fifty and change
a journal of turning fifty and going on

By k.s. lewis

Copyright 2008 by Kurt S. Lewis All Rights Reserved

No part of this book may be reproduced or transmitted in whole or in part in any form or by any means electronic or mechanical, including photocopying, scanning, recording or by an information storage and retrieval system now known or hereafter invented without prior written permission from the publisher, except for the inclusion of brief quotations in a review. This is a work of fiction.

Address inquiries to:

Blue Vagabond Productions
816 Acoma Street #1507
Denver, CO 80204

Cover design by Kurt Lewis

ISBN 978-0-578-00533-1

Sunlight and Shadows
Listen For Home
Listen For Home in black and white
Happiness: A Charlie Travel Adventure Story
Yellow Angels Dancing on a Red Toothbrush: A Charlie Travel Adventure Story

Thank you to all the poets and writers in the world:
your words lit the fire
To those who seek the answers
the simple truth
listen and learn
write to discover
ideas undiscerned
if confused
listen again

Chapter One
Monday, March 20, 2006.

(From Stephan's handwritten journal)

It is 9 a.m. and I am still at home. That has happened more and more lately. At least there is a storm today.

I wish I could write quickly, but perhaps I would just be verbose. The Parkinson's disease may have done me a favor. It is 15 or 16 days until my fiftieth birthday and on that day I have oral arguments in the Court of Appeals. I need to bill incredible hours and the theater development is at a critical point. My girlfriend does dominance sessions in my loft for paying clients and asks how much risk I am taking investing in the theater. And the snow keeps falling.

I slept well last night. I actually controlled my eating. Fiftieth birthday. I was going to marry Mara on my fiftieth birthday, but that was too quick. When we marry we will be hand and fitted glove. It will be forever.

From my seat at the dining table I look out my third story window and see a huge building of condos each for rent for 2000 plus dollars a month on the location where Racine's restaurant used to stand. Racine's was a reason to buy my loft. At least the condos have fancy landscaping.

So many thoughts flash through my mind and suddenly my fingers are wielding the pen with dexterity. Why is that? Do I need just to focus my mind on the fingers? Do I need to meditate? There cannot be a substitute for handwriting a journal.

More coffee. My second cup. Ultimately my writing will define my life. That and the Blues House Theater. However the theater will only be a tool in the writing and in turn the writing will only be the tool to tell stories that change lives. Stories that will amuse and entertain.

The Producers. I guess I shall become Zero Mostel and fund my theater with money given by older women. It will make them happy. I, like Kurt Vonnegut in his last book, will tell you when I am kidding. I am kidding.

I do intend to limit my sexual life to Mara and Mara's command. My mistress, lover, future wife. She calls me her husband and tranny bitch. My guess is that you didn't want to hear that. The concept would kill my parents so I cannot publish a book telling the truth until they die or say its okay. Perhaps I will just say its fiction. The idea of Mara fucking me with a strap-on cock, and me screaming as we both come, won't play in New Town, Kansas.

So I'm kidding, but I'm not. But that is our life and we are happy together and other guys pay Mara to dress them like bitches and whip their ass until they come on her high vinyl boots.

Forty-Nine. Two hundred and forty. Twenty thousand. Age, weight, money in the bank.

Routine: Writing; Reading; Coffee. My Friday mornings with Trevor, a black musician poet-philosopher from eastern Kansas, are inspirational.

I am on page 32 of the Tipping Point, recommended reading by Trevor. I wonder what Levitt the author of Freakonomics would say about the logic, but in any case it is a very interesting marketing book, particularly for the law firm and the theater.

With sleep my mind is a marvelous monster full of creativity—Work out. Sleep. Create. Love Mara. Read. Make a difference.

Headlines in the New York Times: "Plight Deepens for Black Men Studies Warn." The subheading says "Growing Disconnection from the Mainstream."

As I write, I must remember I am Mistress Mara's writer—no one else. What I write I dedicate to her and I acknowledge I crawl on my hands and knees to her feet and suck her toes and clean the bottoms of her feet with my tongue. Odd that strikes me as cat-like behavior. And you did not want to hear that, but I tell you anyway. We love each other.

I serve and she will provide me with inspiration for the remainder of my life. She has a logic that surprises me with its clarity.

Mistress Mara, my wife, may well become a more famous writer than I. I will help guide her and train her natural talent.

Now, she fastens nipple clamps to my tortured pierced nipples. I moan like the bitch she wants me to be for her. She dons the strap on and I suck it –taking it deep. She breathes faster and harder and has me put my head to the floor and my ass in the air and she fucks me and comes herself as I moan—little bitch moans.

Flash to dinner. We talk about our lives, I tell about the joy of diving in the Caribbean. I explain rolling off the boat and opening your eyes to a new world of fish. I want to show her the ocean like she has shown me the joy of submission.

My fiftieth birthday is almost here. Oh my God. Can you believe the day is almost here? I will write my way to fame and fortune. I wish, but I am not kidding.

To tell the truth practicing law is limiting my creativity. That is truth. Right now I do it to pay the bills but it could be much better if I balance the law with writing and theater without stressing myself.

Theater – no it is not theater, it is a concept – a place for convergence of cultures and art forms. That is what we must focus on. And the afternoon plays we develop at the theater will ultimately be our body of work that ends up playing for all time.

Note: Use the afternoon shows to develop work that makes a difference!

So my 50th birthday comes. God. Do you exist? Hell, do I exist? Does fifty, half a century, matter?

11:00 am. I walked into the office and received the cold shoulder treatment from my secretary, Jenny. She disapproves of the theater and coming in late to the office. She's been my secretary for 20 years, but she wants me to focus on the law, drop the theater and work hard.

Driving to work, I spoke to mom and dad. The big news in New Town is that the son-in-law of John Edgar and his daughter are coming back from Saudi Arabia to start a vineyard. My father says flatly that the husband is an Arab. My mom told me how there are other vineyards around Kansas—that it is not new. My parents always talk to me at the same time on two different phones in their house. I cannot remember when they started doing this. I recommend that children speak to their parents this way. There is less jealousy. I still talk to them as I carry heavy bags in from the Jeep through the snow. I love the way they always both get on the telephone with me. Mom thanks me for calling and I tell them, "I love you," and Mom responds, "We love you too." My father grumbles, quietly.

To work now at 11:21 a.m. big day.

Monday

Chapter 1 (continued—originally typed on Stephan's computer).

March 20, 2006

8PM entry.

I have earlier entries for today but I am writing this one at 8pm because I left my notebook at work.

I have to use Dragon because my fingers are balking. So now I am writing with Dragon Speak, a computer software program. Earlier today my fingers started to work but now they are not doing so well. I have gathered my references that are sitting on the bed and under the railing. I sit at the ship's prow, the location that caused me to buy this loft 10 years ago. I dictate to my computer and watch the flat screen where the words appear as I say them, actually there is a few second delay. The Dragon Speak gets more words right than it gets wrong and it is easier for me to write when the Parkinson's disease stops the motor movements in my right hand.

Mara left a few minutes ago. Before she left I showed her the memory quilt that my mother had given me in 1993. Actually my mom and dad gave it to me for Christmas in 1993. I gave Mara the card that my mom had written to me and had her read it to me. It says, "Stephan, December 1993. This is a "memory quilt". Several of the blocks come from pants you wore to high school. The ideas came from Dad and I and Janet. Levin colored in the corn-Jim and Jamie approved the design. Love, Dad and Mom. When Mara finished reading the card she said, "That is wonderful. Maybe they can be my mom and dad too."

Mom, don't read this paragraph. Before Mara came over I dressed the way she likes me dressed. I put on red panties, a calico skirt, a blond wig, my leather collar with rings and high heels. Then we sat on the couch and talked about the Bible and Mara's opinion that Mel Gibson's movie named Passion simply exploited the story of Jesus. Mara told me that when she was in prison she read the Bible three times. When I asked her what she got out of that she asked me if I had ever played the game where you go around the circle whispering a phrase. I said I had. She said the Bible was like that passed down over the centuries. She believes in some of the message but points out that it is contradictory and told by men. She is religious, but not a churchgoer. My dominatrix mistress loves me as a cross-dresser but seriously objects to Mel Gibson's treatment of the story of Christ.

We also talked about her mother, her mother who refuses to talk to me despite the fact that I have supported her daughter. I have paid rent and for operations on Mara's stomach and breasts. Her mother not only doesn't thank me she refuses to talk to me. It is as if I am a bad influence on her daughter. It is very simple, I don't plan on talking to her ever even when she is ready to talk to me, and she will want to talk to me.

These last few years have been a long journey I read from an entry made on Friday, June 9, 2000 at 5:40 a.m.:

"[S]ometimes it is hard to breathe deep. Like now. I have so much that I must get done. So do it. My hands trembled sometimes making it hard to take notes. Is that diabetes or hypoglycemia or too much coffee or too much sugar or pending nervous breakdown or bad shoulder or out of shape or carpal tunnel or what?"

I had no clue that it was Parkinson's disease. I thought it was my shoulder and my finger. In fact, it was an entire year before I found out that it was Parkinson's.

So I turn 50 in a few days. April 3, 2006 I shall be half a century old engaged to a girl who is 24. Incredible. Not only is she 24 but she is gorgeous and very smart. Actually, I think she will become a writer. She says she wants to something for troubled kids because that's what she was and she ended up in prison. She made me laugh tonight when she said, "Did you know I was a certified janitor?" Laughing I said, no way. But she had become a certified janitor in prison. She also told a story about the preacher who came to teach them in prison and how that preacher had left his family and his parish to meet with a girl from an Internet connection. How that preacher had been put in prison because he had hurt the four-year-old daughter of the girl. Mara said, "He must have shaken that four-year-old like a rag doll to inflict the brain damage they said occurred." So she used that example and said to me, "I'm not a churchgoing person."

She also talked about parents who let kids have BB guns and how she opposes that. We had a wonderful conversation holding hands. It was like we were two love struck kids.

So there is the Mara talks to me about kids and BB guns and national policy. Then there is a Mara who is my dominatrix mistress who pulls on the nipple clamps until I scream in pain. She makes me masturbate in front of her wearing the nipple clamps until I come and then she makes me lick the floor clean. We are both freaky together.

My ex-girlfriend would say I'm brainwashed and I would say I am in love. Engaged to be married. Mara told me that if I died she would have to beat me back to life.

I remember the guy who takes care of the clubhouse at Bear Creek. He is very old but still in very good shape physically and mentally. My client Jimmy Dice asked him how he stayed so fit and the fellow said, "a young wife."

It is ten PM. I am going to bed now.

Chapter Two
March 21, 2006. 5am.

So many thoughts run through my mind about my first fifty years, actually my first 49 years and 350 days or thereabouts. I am typing this morning and I think about the day I was diagnosed with Parkinson's disease. The doctor, I cannot remember her name, said, you will always remember this day. She was right. I remember that day and the day before when I made Rachel, my ex-girlfriend, mad, because I delayed starting home from Kansas to play one-on-one basketball with my nephew Levin. I won even with a few unexpected air balls. It was the last time I played basketball with him. He grew up and played some decent high school basketball and I was diagnosed with Parkinson's, my doctor prescribed Mirapex, a dopamine agonist, and my life changed.

In between then and now I was a large part of winning a multi-million dollar verdict for a client, I began producing plays, worked on two theaters that closed and now am working on my dream theater. In between I have met thousands of people, some who stand out as good some as bad, and most as in-between. My play Blue Vagabond was produced and received critical acclaim. And for those first few years I operated in a mental fog. My lack of sustained writing evidences that fog. I almost died on the highway several times due to falling asleep and my ex-girlfriend left me due to the Parkinsonian-Mirapex related symptoms of sleepiness, addictive behavior and work. I laugh, that made me think of ex-law partners over the years. My favorites are the characters. Ron Raily is my favorite, perhaps because he fought and is still fighting the effects of Polio. I hear he read poetry at the Mercury Café where I now hang out – with a poet Trevor Pale who has become my best male friend. Ron wore his hair long and wore outrageous suits; he had a Jim Carrey orange suit, represented the gambling industry and published a book of poetry. I wish I had read it. Now I don't know where to find it.

Looking back is amusing, but I am not done with life. Trevor and I get together every Friday morning and talk about art and the theater and a poet's night at the Blues House. If I am in Chicago this Friday we will get together on Saturday morning. Now it is 5:39 AM. I shall lay down for a moment or two or shall I go work out? I cannot believe I wasted so much writing time playing online scrabble and looking at naked women on cam and profiles of people. I, like the Blue Vagabond, was searching for someone or something. I found Mara in real life and not on the internet and the two of us have lived far more of life than you can imagine Mom. Mara wants to meet you and I want you to meet her. It is imperative that it happen because she is the love of my life. She needs a Mom like you and I hope you and Dad come on the train to visit for my fiftieth birthday or thereabouts as you said you might.

The story of the Blue Vagabond circles and he discovers that his essence was that he told stories that had truth in them. Oh my god. I realize I have just lived the story of the Blue Vagabond in real life and that I am a storyteller. How could I have missed this? Perhaps I will be like all those other Mirapex crazed persons who spent their fortunes on addictive behaviors---sue the manufacturer. Just kidding. They might cutoff the Mirapex I am still taking. Okay now it is 5:55am and I will go work out at the Matrix, a gym a block away. Amazing that I typed this entire entry.

Okay so I haven't gone yet. I put on my running clothes, poked my nose outside and realized that it is still snowing. I made coffee and consider whether to run in the cold or go one block in the cold to the Matrix or stay in and work out with my stationary bike or weights. I opened the upper shade on my huge West window and I see gray clouds obscuring the mountains completely. There are only a few flakes of snow, steam from my neighbor's vents on their roof. I can see down into their loft but I rarely look, I like the view to the West over their rounded green metal roof. In the past, I have drawn the classic architecture of West High and its bell tower.

I cannot remember the name of the girl who greeted me so warmly at the Tattered Cover book store on Saturday night when I bought The Tipping Game, The New York Times Manual of Style and Usage, the Language of the Blues, and The Copywriter's Handbook. I had bought a grape soda and Danish which I balanced precariously on my stack of books. I saw this couple sitting there, the woman was very attractive and the guy a bit dumpy and I looked for an open table. I did not recognize her at all but she went, "Stepppppphhhhhhan" and got up and hugged me after I set my stack down. I remembered when I last saw her, at Kathy's party which she told I was in September of last year. She had been telling this guy about the Blues House Theater next to the Mercury Café and poof I had appeared.

How embarrassing to be introduced to Brin, she playfully called him Briney, and not remember the name of the person who hugs me in recognition. I will have to figure out her name. I figured out the name of the banker whose name I was trying to remember the other day, Francine Deller. She was driven to nail forgers and embezzlers to the wall, but she retained her sense of humor into her seventies.

I want to invite blues bands into the Blues House Theater. Find them and invite them and call it the Blues night at the Blues House. Perhaps Thursday nights after the early show. Why? Because I love the blues and I will write a song called The Lawyer Blues. Now work out!!!!!

Oh I have to invite William Shatner to visit too. His portrayal of a lawyer on Boston Legal at times makes me cry in recognition and sympathy for his character. It is the best acting I have ever seen him do.

So age fifty comes in a few days. How many? Hmmm. When will I finish the theater? I cannot wait but will it happen. Christ I need to bill some hours to pay the bills. And I have to meet the general contractor at 10AM today. Get going.

Chapter Three
March 22, 2006

I sit in my office overlooking the confluence between the Platte River and Cherry Creek and consider fifty years of life. The phone rings. Ironic. Typical. Who in my office would consider the implications of life I consider? The young associates. Perhaps Janice. Probably Janice. Jenny's life swirls about her: kids; sick mother, house in the suburbs, boss who doesn't focus on work (me).

Rumpole comes to mind. The storyteller who lived or lives from case to case in the Old Bailey. Who was the author? John Mortimer. I would like to meet John Mortimer and ask him about how it happened.

Fifty arrives. The thought of changing –the phone rings again—this time an old not-so-close friend, Don Zebner calling about baseball tickets. I still have two seats behind home plate. Maybe this year I will go there and write. Baseball, I had a long conversation with Barry, a client who saw and loved the Blue Vagabond and saw Cowgirls.

11 Am. I have not billed time yet today. Yet I have written. My fingers are working this morning.

Do you suppose the partner I have who speaks in grunts when I pass him in the hall would read a poem to his lover? I smile. I amuse myself today.

I spoke to Rita Tabor who said she missed our long philosophical conversations. She started painting my house and dedicated a book she wrote to me.

Tonight at the Denver Public Library the mayor is hosting the induction of the new Denver poet laureate. I plan to go.

Looking at an old notebook I see I wrote on 12/9/2000: "I'm an unshaved fat orca with bad breath." I drew a line and wrote "Title of a Play." I was twenty pounds overweight in 2000. I could not have dreamed that I would be 240 pounds in 2006.

I also wrote: "170 CLTM create, condition, Alive, Rachel, Listen, try the cases, In the moment. Condition. Create. Meditate."

I wrote, "I need to spend the rest of my life writing and conditioning...."

Now, five years later I am turning fifty. Here I am.

Last night. Last night. Yesterday I hosted my business planning class after we visited the Denver Public library. Then at 1 am Mistress went with me to see a transsexual named Bren who had me suck her cock and then she fucked me harder than I have ever been fucked in my life. I am a slut for Mistress, a sexual playboy.

All that wiped out the thoughts of a day in which I ran ten minutes on the treadmill with my heart beat at 169-170 and in which I had a long wonderful conversation with Trevor Pale in the morning and a day in which the law firm celebrated Jenny's 41st birthday by ordering from the Italian place Magana's. I just got off the phone with Trevor who is going wild with poetry and theater ideas.

The grim reality of today is not enough work this month, not enough money to do the theater and I am stressed due to not being at work and the very thing that I should be doing, writing, is causing the stress. It is time for change and the theater will provide that change. That and the writing. I am turning fifty with a twenty-four year old dominatrix girl friend, a Renaissance man poet as my best friend, and the experience to actually make amazing things happen. So will we get the theater built? Yes. Will Mara and I get married? Yes.

Will this story have a happy ending? Fifty is coming. I have a huge oral argument on April 3, 2006. I want Mara to see it. Now I must go but I will find stories of this day.

1:35 PM

(Written in Stephan's small black note book)

Playing hooky now. I came home because I have gas cause I ate too many of the pinto beans I cooked up in the crock pot. They are cleaning out my system though. Shane Heitman, my law partner, turns fifty tomorrow. How will he react? One thing of which I am certain. He does not know the feeling I have right now of the inability to write down the words. Another thing of which I am certain, he is not writing a book about turning fifty.

(The following was typed on Stephan's computer that he named Sajina after one of his fictional characters)

The Transsexual named Bren had the tightest butt muscles. She, or is it he, said she had just got back from working out. As I was leaving she showed me her silver crowns that she had won and a picture of her looking like Selena. Bren is Hispanic with a big smile, a scorpion tattoo in the middle of her stomach just above the belly button, and a pierced tongue. It was fun frolicking naked in bed with her.

Am I really turning fifty? I am just learning how to live. Or at least some variety has appeared in my life. Music, I need music while I write, because I am writing for my dinner. Lol. I know what Lol means—laughing out loud. I started a blog a few weeks ago. That began the resurrection of my scribbling. Shall I quit the law and write, run a theater and beg for money. First things first get the theater built. Once I have the theater built I have a way to make money other than the law. The third way is to write, but I cannot count on books, at least not yet.

I have been saying to myself over and over again, "I have to make my weaknesses my strengths. Thus I must organize my life down to the tacks in the sheets covering up the desk in the living room. One of which I accidently pulled out and stepped on Sunday. My foot bled profusely and I did not get a tetanus shot.

Dr. John's Anutha Zone is playing. New Orleans oozes from his words and I realize I must get out of the office and make my money in the streets, become a lawyer dropout, a mystic writer, an artist making a difference.

While looking at the Ralph Steadman drawings in Hunter Thompson's Fear and Loathing in Las Vegas that I loaned to Sam to read, I predict that in the end I will be the client. Oh my god there are 13 days, counting today before I turn fifty. Thirteen days to examine the first half century of my life. Thirteen days to find answers to life. Thirteen days before the counter clicks and clatters and stops at fifty.

Speaking to Rita today I realized that I inspire people to create and I am the leader. Others probably scoff and say I am indecisive, but what leader has not had indecision in his or her life. I have learned so much and now I must marshal that knowledge into an incredible transformation. At fifty, the clock shall stop and I shall blossom into me.

Cell phones. Voice mail sorry your mailbox is full. Messages from Sam, Mara, Jay from Miami who wants to fuck Mara, another message from Mara, Greg who has liver cancer and has to start chemo soon, Mara again, Jack calling about taxes for last year which is killing me, Jackie calling about teaching a class for acting for lawyers – there is another source of income hopefully—Jack again who saved the theater by putting Greg and me back together, Luke the artist guy who will help coordinate the art in Blues House, the client whose case is up for argument on April 3—I suppose the climax of this narrative, Rachel calling to thank me for getting her the gig at the coffee shop near the theater, Mara who tells me she loves me, Trevor confirming a meeting. Trevor inviting me to a family barbecue. Wayne from Rocky Horror Picture Show called concerning their show. Xavier called, he is the dance teacher that is working with us. Rachel called wanting me to come over and watch the movie Crash. Trevor called and I went to the barbecue. Wayne confirming we needed 40 people a night to cover licensing costs for Rocky Horror. Sam calling to make sure I made it to a firm meeting. Rachel calling to say Tessa wants to buy my truck by making payments. I laughed. Rachel again saying that she thought I was ordered not to call her back. Janie calling about joining our firm as an intellectual property attorney. She is a writer too!!!!

The woman who cleans my house calling to verify cleaning my house. She is from the Philippines. That reminds me that Shane Heitman grew up in the Philippines and other places and may have stories to tell about different places. Then a message from my new hair stylist. She said she hoped my hair is growing fast so she can hear about the theater. Message from a guy about being the general contractor for the theater. And then Rachel called to remind me to watch Boston Legal. So those are the people calling me the past few weeks.

Now I am going to the library to meet Trevor and to attend part of the induction of the new poet laureate of Denver. Afterwards it seemed the words of Poet Laureate and the Mayor applied to us.

9PM

Mara and I just ate a wonderful dinner at Bambino's. She looks very much like Britney Spears only much smarter and I love just holding her hand at dinner. It is hard to think of her as a bank robber, a felon and smuggling pot into prison in her pussy. She said she wants to take psychology classes, perhaps because of all the therapists she has seen.

I will have to write more but now I am going to bed.

Chapter Four.
March 23, 2006

Ten minutes after midnight and I am writing again. I woke up at 11:30 p.m. and grabbed a bunch of books and through them on the ground beneath my feet where I sit in the ugly green chair now covered by the Mexican blanket that used to be on the couch, my horse blanket, the memory quilt given to me by my mother and father and an eggplant colored towel. While pulling out the books I found what I have been looking for earlier today, Rita Tabor's book, "Airline Fever." She wrote in the forward to the book, "For Stephan, you believe in me. You've always supported and pushed me towards my goals. You made me focus. You continually reminded me that everyone "starts" somewhere. I think you for everything you've given, loaned and sold to me."

Previously, I had begun to read Rita's book that this time I started to read it and laughed out loud because I could hear her voice talking to me. She is truly a writer. She has a unique voice.

Am I being self-indulgent in writing this book? Will my actress friend Jackie read the scribbles and snort in derision? Will I snort in derision when I read it? Will these words be a fizzled coming out party that nobody reads but everybody knows about? Will I regret the fuck out of this? Will I write the rest of my life in questions?

May I be as bold as Rita has been. What a gutsy woman she is!

So Trevor and I am a pair. We went together to listen to the induction of the poet laureate and now I forget his name again just as I can't remember the name of the woman who hugged me and at the Tattered Cover bookstore on Saturday night. Hopefully her name comes to me soon. I am seriously waiting for the name to appear on my tongue.

I suppose I could edit out the embarrassing parts, but then what the fuck would it be? Fiction?

I'm writing this chapter using Dragon Speak, training the program as I go. Sometimes the Dragon speaks on its own. Like I have told others, the dragon is creative.

So there is some tension in this narrative. On April 3, 2006 I will argue an appeal, which, if I win, could change my life. The next few days I must prepare for that argument and on Monday I present the argument to my clients who are difficult, so difficult that they did not talk to me for weeks after we filed the appellate brief because they didn't feel they had enough opportunity to make corrections. Since then they have decided that the brief was pretty well written after all. This Friday, the opposition in the Chicago case I am working on will be filing a summary judgment brief. That too will govern my life. In addition, I need to finish the business plan for the theater and raise money.

My breath shortens as I think of the things to be done. Oh, and there's taxes in addition. Damn. Mara is going to Las Vegas to have her photo shoot on March 31. I'm not going or am I? Maybe I will. Just maybe I will. I need to be prepared for the arguments in advance. Las Vegas March 31. I think I will go.

Mara is the important thing in my life and what is best about her is she cares about me and the theater. We talked about hiking and transsexuals during dinner. We connect on many levels and I love her beyond belief. I have to lose weight because I cannot afford to lose her. I want to present my best self to her. When I am conditioned not only am I more attractive, but I am also more creative. It is 12:56 am on March 23, 2006. I turn 50 on April 3. Time is short. Life is short. As Trevor said today, or actually yesterday, when referring to building the theater, "Enjoy the ride!"

I need to find the quotes by Tennessee Williams about writing. My barren time is over. During that time I played many games of

Scrabble online certainly over 1000 games. I think it improved my vocabulary and my thinking. There was a purpose in it was to refill the well of creativity which has been done.

What books did I pull from the shelves? General Psychiatry to study my quirks; Nietzsche to study my philosophy; Zapatismo, to study the philosophy of another client, Brandon Pearson, who has invited me to help put in fence posts in Southern Colorado. It is odd to think I have a client who has land in Wyoming that has a missile silo in which they are going to test rockets. I've agreed to show up on the Fourth of July in Wyoming at the missile silo. I also have a client whose graphic artist is Ralph Steadman who did the artwork for Fear and Loathing in Las Vegas. I will not stop practicing law. Practice of law makes many things possible for me so stopping would simply be stupidity. That much is clear. The theater will also generate an enormous group of clients.

The Three Musketeers----Greg, Jack, Stephan and Trevor is d'Artagnan. Actually, Trevor said it best, "We have to collect our family."

Dragon speak helps me enunciate and thus will help me argue m appeal. Now it is 1:20 Am. I Also Chose "The Fool's Progress an Honest Novel" by Edward Abbey, one my favorite novels if indeed it is a novel. I chose "The Blue Knight" due to its compelling story. I chose Sex in the City because it is fun. There is an entertainment law textbook that I pulled out and finally, "Mindfulness." I almost forgot a little book I pulled out named, "don't sweat the small stuff." Oops, there were a few books covered by the blanket, "Care of the Soul" that reminds me of Kate Narcissi who had and probably still has big hair and a fiery temperament. The Great Thoughts. A Hundred Verses from Old Japan. And most importantly, Abbey's "One Life at a Time, Please." In "One Life" Abbey says it is the writer's duty to tell the truth. Kurt Vonnegut said that he wrote the book "Slaughterhouse Five" when he finally understood that he just needed to tell the truth. War. Death and dying in Iraq. Youngsters dying. We should not allow youngsters to fight our wars. If a leader orders people to go to war it should be required that he is on the frontline.

The last book is Steve Martin's "Picasso at the Lapin Agile." Wonderful writing by Steve Martin. One more. The Mexicans, a personal portrait of a people of a people. And of course I started reading Airline Fever by Rita Tabor. Now it is 1:45 am and I must go back to sleep. There is so little time, but on the other hand, as Trevor said, "Enjoy the ride."

10:23 AM. Yesterday afternoon, Trevor and I attended the induction of the poet Laureate of Denver and the mayor John Hickenlooper introduced Chis Ransick as the new poet laureate. The mayor announced a new initiative to put poetry on RTD. Then Chris and the mayor talked about how important it was to include poetry in the cultural life of the city and in the schools. Trevor kept nudging me because it sounded as if the Mayor and Chris Ransick had been listening to us plan Blues House future. Afterwards we had coffee and I realized that we need to train poets to go out into the schools and Blues House will be a place for the results of that training applied to the schools.

Today is the fiftieth birthday for Shane, my law partner. He works with his door closed and I wonder if he has even thought about his life, his friends, his experiences and his future—other than making money practicing law?

2:00 PM. I saw Shane in the restroom, he was standing front of the urinal and I asked, "How does it feel?" He had just turned fifty. He said, "It feels strange to be on the second half of a century. It is like when our parents and grandparents told us about World War I and World War II. Now we tell our kids about the fifties and sixties—well actually the sixties and seventies.

I am sitting at the restaurant near our office called Shakespeare in a building with a huge "For Lease" sign on it. I listen to jazz music and the clack of pool balls and eat a large Cobb Salad with honey-mustard dressing. There are twenty or more pool tables on either side of a ship's bridge with tables, bar and piano.

Chapter Five
March 24, 2006.

12:30 pm. This morning I was overwhelmed with phone calls and stuff. I met with Trevor this morning after getting very little sleep last night. Now it takes me thirty minutes to compose a few line email. I go to sleep and the keys get stuck on a letter lllllllllllllllllllllllllllllllll or sssssssssssssssssssssssss sssssssssssssssssssssssssssssssssss sssssssssssssssssssssssssssssssssssssssssssssssssssss. It can go for many lines. I have to wake up and delete the run-on rows of letters. I worry that I will send out something that way. Yesterday, I was overwhelmed by a spate of telephone calls. I had worked out in the morning with a run walk around Cheeseman Park with my trainer who is developing an intervention plan to combat my Parkinson's disabilities. Then I worked out at the Matrix for another hour and got myself down to 235 but last night blew some of that gain in conditioning due to eating and lack of sleep.

4:30pm. Damn. So much is happening I cannot even begin to scribble all of it. The owner of the space on Welton is interested in having us assume the debt with the city. Amazing. We are designing a theater which will work synergistically with the coffee shop. What is going to happen?

Without sleep I feel ineffective and fat. I suppose I am fat. I made a clay figure of a fat man avoiding a coffin. That image sticks in my mind right now. I am working on the business plan and trying to prepare for the arguments in the Court of Appeals.

Chapter Six
March 25, 2006

Yesterday I felt like I threw myself under a car and died and was still trying to function. Now at 4AM I am awake and alive. On days like yesterday I should just go back to bed and try to sleep. I miss so much of life on a day like yesterday. What did I miss?

The most entertaining event contest included the meeting between the former owners of Muddy's coffee shop with Greg, Trevor and me. Greg and Trevor clash on many subjects, Trevor exudes optimism about life and Greg seems a cynic, but they agree on building a theater with enthusiasm and love. Greg dislikes the poetry scene; Trevor revels in it. However, Greg loves Maya Angelo and Trevor mentored under her.

I could not help but notice the intensity of Greg and Trevor and when Greg described some of his off-beat music lyric projects, Trevor, the musician, suggested they spend some quality time together away from others.

So it is almost 5AM. I want to live with Mara as husband and wife. We need to embrace as we go to sleep. I need to get my body in perfect shape at 175-180 lbs. for Mara. So I must run this morning. As I say that I also realize that I must intensely prepare for the court of appeals arguments.

I brought my non-legal books home from the office yesterday after Cheryl and Jenny packed them off my shelves and commandeered my shelves for case notebooks. The Chicago case is still alive which means I have substantial paying work for the next few months.

Creativity. Yesterday morning I had my weekly Friday meeting with Trevor and looked out the window of the coffee shop next to the theater and saw on the window of the building across the street the word, "Creativity." I am going to incorporate the location of the theater into the business plan. The business plan should be finished this weekend in draft.

Right now I am going to build the bookcases that I bought a week ago and brought home from Office Depot yesterday. I need my books on the shelves. I write standing up typing in the kitchen. When I finish the shelves and fill them with books I will write on the dining room table next to the books.

I have a desire to worship Mistress Mara's body and legs and breasts and toes and feet right this moment. I delight in the thought of her and build the bookcases. I can feel her whip on my ass and her toes entwined in the chain of my nipple clamps. She pulls not so lightly on the chain with her toes. I moan and she smiles and asks, "Who owns you?" I say, "You own me Mistress. Mistress Mara owns me." And then she kneels in front of me and focuses her intense brown eyes in mine and says, "I own you forever. Now masturbate your cock for me. Who owns that cock?" I say, "You do Mistress. I love you." I can feel the moment now because it happened. Is there such a thing as coming out as a Mistress and a Slave? We may find out.

I think of Mara calling me last night and telling me good night and that she loves me dearly and I love her. I enjoy every moment we spend together and my mind goes to Racine's where at the very moment that I broke up with her I knew I loved her and was making a mistake. The only excuse I have is that I did not believe she loved me. Now I do believe. I know and I do not question that love. We are engaged for marriage and I want that to happen.

Chapter Seven
March 26, 2006. 8:06AM.

I fully intended to write more yesterday but the day gathered momentum and then accelerated out of my grasp. I finished the building the two five-shelf bookcases and filled them with books, VHS movies and DVD movies. Quite an array of stories to draw on for inspiration and entertainment. Sometimes I believe I could just hole up here in my loft and create my way out of debt. Is that a dream? I will never know unless I try.

What do I have to do today? Don't think about that yet, just write. I have the Dragon Speak program ready but I have not turned it on yet and I am laboriously typing out the words. The left hand works fine, but the right slows the typing process immensely. Perhaps there is some rehab I can do?

White and Strunk's The Elements of Style says to place the emphatic words at the end of the sentence. Have I ever read White and Strunk cover to cover? I bought the New York Times Manual of Style last week when I saw the girl whose name I could not remember. It seems as if she wrote her phone number and address for me somewhere when we saw each other at the party, but I have not looked hard because I am owned by Mara, my Mistress. Her tattoo is on my back. She branded me not long after we got back together last summer.

I type on Sajina and my fingers have become more deft. I set up on the dining room table which is in the corner near the two new bookcases. Last night at three in the morning when I could not sleep I brought the Yamaha keyboard downstairs and set it up by the bookcase on the West wall. Now I can open the shade on my back door and look out to the west and play music or type or use the keyboard as a midi.

I intensely need Mistress now. I need her. Yesterday she did not call until late in the day and I was distraught wondering if she was abandoning me or if the whole relationship was just based upon the thousands and thousands of dollars I have given her or spent on her. But I sit here in my Victoria Secret panties that she got for me after she had me try them on with her in the Victoria Secret dressing room at the 16th Street Mall. She told me to come in the dressing room with her and strip and then she had me try on panties. These say "Tease Me" on the front.

And now I am Mistress Mara's bitch. I went to the bathroom and put on my red lipstick and blond wig and now I have high heels on. I am not supposed to touch my cock. I put on her nipple clamps and I have to call her now and ask permission to stroke my cock. Mistress I need you. But the call is of no use because her messages are full. This is frustrating. How will all of this turn out? Will we be married or does she string me along for the money? I smile. I am not going to worry about this now. Mara owns me and I love her. When she has me suck her strap on cock it is real, the question remains, how will our relationship evolve? She says and I say it is forever. That is what it will be; there is no room for doubts.

toxic_alternative (3/22/2006 12:03:34 AM): i switched computers

marasecret (3/22/2006 12:03:50 AM): coolhow r u

toxic_alternative (3/22/2006 12:04:11 AM): it still doesnt work

toxic_alternative (3/22/2006 12:04:14 AM): damn

toxic_alternative (3/22/2006 12:04:24 AM): i will go on alt

marasecret (3/22/2006 12:04:47 AM): go on alt

toxic_alternative (3/22/2006 12:05:02 AM): did u find someone to fuck ur bitch?

marasecret (3/22/2006 12:05:17 AM): not yet

marasecret (3/22/2006 12:06:40 AM): did u get onaalt?

toxic_alternative (3/22/2006 12:07:19 AM): i am on trying to load cam maybe i switch cams

marasecret (3/22/2006 12:09:29 AM): tryit

marasecret (3/22/2006 12:12:37 AM): is it working

toxic_alternative (3/22/2006 12:15:24 AM): not yet just a secd

marasecret (3/22/2006 12:21:46 AM): resend it6

toxic_alternative (3/22/2006 12:23:36 AM): it is not working

marasecret (3/22/2006 12:24:59 AM): i know pisses me off

toxic_alternative (3/22/2006 12:25:08 AM): changing internet connections

toxic_alternative (3/22/2006 12:26:08 AM): do u have msn messenger?

marasecret (3/22/2006 12:26:15 AM): nope

marasecret (3/22/2006 12:26:53 AM): grrrrrrrrr

toxic_alternative (3/22/2006 12:27:23 AM): i think the cam issue is on ur side have u tried restarting?

marasecret (3/22/2006 12:30:03 AM): i can see alt cams

marasecret (3/22/2006 12:30:08 AM): yes i restarted

toxic_alternative (3/22/2006 12:30:14 AM): k

marasecret (3/22/2006 12:30:19 AM): u need to b fucked 4 me

marasecret (3/22/2006 12:30:27 AM): http://www.eros-denver.com/sections/tvts.htm

toxic_alternative (3/22/2006 12:30:30 AM): mmmm

marasecret (3/22/2006 12:31:38 AM): ulike her?

toxic_alternative (3/22/2006 12:32:04 AM): i have to go separately which one

toxic_alternative (3/22/2006 12:32:54 AM): i am there but i dont know which one

marasecret (3/22/2006 12:33:25 AM): VALERIA

marasecret (3/22/2006 12:33:31 AM): OR ALLANAH

marasecret (3/22/2006 12:33:47 AM): TOMMORROW

marasecret (3/22/2006 12:33:54 AM): EARLY LIKE 4PM?

toxic_alternative (3/22/2006 12:34:42 AM): shall i call valeriie and have u listen to me get fucked tonight

marasecret (3/22/2006 12:35:18 AM): YES

toxic_alternative (3/22/2006 12:36:08 AM): calling

toxic_alternative (3/22/2006 12:37:35 AM): message

marasecret (3/22/2006 12:37:45 AM): MAKE AN APPT TOMMORROW

toxic_alternative (3/22/2006 12:37:53 AM): ok

marasecret (3/22/2006 12:37:59 AM): CALL ALLANAH

toxic_alternative (3/22/2006 12:39:01 AM): does she have #

toxic_alternative (3/22/2006 12:39:42 AM): what do u think of brandy

marasecret (3/22/2006 12:41:07 AM): leave the credit card there for me tommor for flight and hotel

marasecret (3/22/2006 12:41:10 AM): call her

toxic_alternative (3/22/2006 12:41:32 AM): calling

toxic_alternative (3/22/2006 12:43:56 AM): 20 min at 13th and colo incall

marasecret (3/22/2006 12:43:58 AM): 82 917 239-3713 call raquel

marasecret (3/22/2006 12:44:18 AM): i wanna b there?

toxic_alternative (3/22/2006 12:44:30 AM): u coming ?

marasecret (3/22/2006 12:44:44 AM): lol not tonite you can go

toxic_alternative (3/22/2006 12:45:09 AM): she is local

marasecret (3/22/2006 12:45:27 AM): try raquel tho i like her better maybe she can come to the loft tommorrow

toxic_alternative (3/22/2006 12:45:31 AM): if she is good then mmmm

marasecret (3/22/2006 12:45:52 AM): raquel isnt local but rubi is marasecret (3/22/2006 12:46:03 AM): call that number

toxic_alternative (3/22/2006 12:46:31 AM): Mistress may i check out brandy?

marasecret (3/22/2006 12:46:46 AM): yes call that number tho k

marasecret (3/22/2006 12:46:50 AM): now

toxic_alternative (3/22/2006 12:46:56 AM): which one

marasecret (3/22/2006 12:47:07 AM): t82 917 200-3000

toxic_alternative (3/22/2006 12:47:17 AM): who?

marasecret (3/22/2006 12:47:59 AM): 917 200 3000 raquel

marasecret (3/22/2006 12:48:10 AM): then u can go see rubi

toxic_alternative (3/22/2006 12:49:17 AM): calling

toxic_alternative (3/22/2006 12:50:22 AM): she said half our notice exit 215 off i-25

marasecret (3/22/2006 12:50:39 AM): HUH

marasecret (3/22/2006 12:50:41 AM): ???

toxic_alternative (3/22/2006 12:50:46 AM): strange

marasecret (3/22/2006 12:51:05 AM): ok go see brandy k

toxic_alternative (3/22/2006 12:51:27 AM): k

marasecret (3/22/2006 12:51:34 AM): leave the card for me in the morning k

toxic_alternative (3/22/2006 12:51:56 AM): k

marasecret (3/22/2006 12:52:01 AM): call me when your done.... Ur gonna go get fucked for me right

toxic_alternative (3/22/2006 12:52:11 AM): yes Mistress

toxic_alternative (3/22/2006 12:52:29 AM): does that please u

marasecret (3/22/2006 12:52:46 AM): yes alot

toxic_alternative (3/22/2006 12:52:58 AM): i will call on the way

marasecret (3/22/2006 12:54:28 AM): call afterward k

It is damning and interesting that you can call up all your old conversations on yahoo if you make the right settings.

Distracted again. Rachel called and invited me to Racine's. I reluctantly agreed to go. I have not been there since the incident with Mara where I had Rachel whisk away the Cherokee. Oddly, or ironically I am driving the Cherokee today because I switched with Cheryl who had been driving it. Ok. I will be back shortly and I will continue writing, I will work out hard and I will prepare for the court of appeals arguments and I will work on the business plan and I will work on the joint venture with the retailers next to the theater to make the purchase of the retail space happen. The theater may be how I support myself. I can lower my overhead by quitting the law firm and focusing on the theater. Hmmm. I can still practice law with a low overhead. Interesting but not yet.

Fifty approaches. How many days now? Eight days counting today. I feel a huge change approaching.

5PM. I still haven't done any work today and I am supposed to make a presentation tomorrow. Instead I have been distracted by ex-girlfriend's, taking sexy cross-dressing pictures for my current girlfriend and oddly I can type really well right now. What I haven't done is waste time playing online scrabble or even by being online chatting. Rachel took me to the store where we got the Magnesium relaxant and I got two bottles. Hopefully that leads to good sleep. At Racine's I ate only one half of a Cobb salad so perhaps my days of gluttony are over. Rachel and I worked on the lyrics of a song she had created. "I'm a slow train wreck" is the title. I came up with lots of alternatives for her lyrics and we will see how it all comes out.

I plan on working out yet today. I told my trainer in an email that I could pay for my next round of sessions when she emailed me saying she did not know how her finances would work without it. Christ I am the supporter of many. Greg needs money. Jack needs money and the only thing that may save me is buying the theater.

I met with the retailers last night at 7:30 at a coffee shop and we discussed the purchase of the retail space. They are all for it and I need to draft the documents to make it happen. That and draft the business plan. All of a sudden though I can type and it is time to work on the business plan and this journal. Who knows when the fingers will stop working?

Yesterday I also met with Dave Zebner who is going to help with the financial analysis of the theater. Actually I had dinner with him and his wife at Pingo's Pizza and we divided the baseball tickets. I need to deliver tickets to my ex-wife, who has gotten all her money from me already.

Rachel cannot get a job, Mara spends money like there is an unending flow and there are assorted others that see me as the source of riches. Me, I am one half million dollars in debt with assets of 800,000. I need to write my way out of the trap and make zero balances come to pass.

Law helps immensely. Do not give it up. But I have to start paying substantial taxes. I have received 56,000 in distributions this year already. I have no credit card debt, but I have to pay taxes and I may get killed soon. Next problem is raising money for the theater. Jimmy Dice volunteered $50,000 the day after I call. I called my farm banker and he will need to do an appraisal before he can advance any more money, but that is a source. Land prices are close to 3000 an acre and the Landers quarter could have a pivot on it. That adds up to 480,000 dollars is that right? Hmmm. Perhaps I should have him get the appraisal.

I have to keep clients. I have to get the work done. Last year I lost several good clients due to my failure to get stuff done quickly and failure to be aggressive in litigation. The Parkinson's disease and the drugs are directly responsible but I can help myself by getting in physical shape.

Back from a run/walk.

>Time rolls relentlessly
>Fingers stiffen uncontrollably
>Eyes wrinkle imperceptibly.
>The path around the park.
>Lengthens every year
>Hills grow steeper
>Making my feet plod deeper
>Into the dust and mud
>As I run that path
>Around the park.
>Faces long known disappear
>Or wrinkle in despair
>But rocks are rocks
>And trees are trees
>Blossoming soft spring leaves.
>Grass is grass
>And sun is sun.
>Someday I shall be the rocks
>the trees the sun
>Someday I shall be the dust beneath your feet
>And then the rain shall cool the sun
>Turning me to mud
>That squishes between your toes.
>So when my face disappears
>Remember me when you run
>That dusty path around the park.

Checkmate.

A pawn hustles the night watch woman
hoping the King has lost his Queen,
The Bishop takes a nun for a knight
and sacrifices his diagonal life,
Queens trade pawns for pawns
and avoid the Knights,
Rooks observe and wait their turn,
Reverie invades my mind
putting me out of sweet time,
The whistle blows,
the chime chimes twelve
the locks are loosed
And the dogs of war play hell
on their toes of gold made by Dell
Death come fast to those who sleep
while politicos heap
False truths upon false hopes
to open the doors of war.
And suddenly.
Sickeningly.
It's not a game anymore.
Sons dying, mothers crying, pawns we are,
Blood flows and bodies stack in rows
When did the game end and this killing begin?
Behead the pawn, stab the knight,

grenades are now the fight,
And the king sees nothing,
Always blinded
by the light of citizens votes.
Now we know the right,
 we were wrong.

Chapter Eight
March 28, 2006

    5:21 a.m. I have read about the man condemned to death because he converted from Islam to Christianity. He disappeared after he was released from an Afghan prison. Prosecutors released him on the grounds he was mentally unfit to stand trial.

    As I read this story on the internet I ate, with trembling fingers, a lettuce, tomato and avocado salad with poppy seed dressing. I woke earlier feeling poetic but the computer took so long to load that I lost some of that feeling. Best I scribble the words, but that is not so easy with Parkinson's disease. However, I am typing these words and I will break to take drugs so the typing becomes easier.

    Time limits all. Time and mortality limit all human endeavors. Mortality is a function of time with a different unknown variable for each human. Foreseen death denied limits the mind's creations as much as the unknown. So crystal balls and cancer have much in common.

    Body and mind exhausted, I failed to write yesterday. Last night I slept and dreamed awakening only to call Mara because I had not heard her call as she said she would do when she arrived home.

    The clock says 5:58 a. m. It is almost time for my morning "run." Workouts are as essential as writing, as essential as friends, as essential as a fire on a cold snowy day in the mountains. Without workouts I freeze into a person unknown to me.

    Yesterday I returned Cabaret,
The movie that helped me understand

My mistress

Who loves me so.

I love her unconditionally

No matter she plays untraditionally

With me

And others who adore her

All that matters

Love from me to her

And her to me

I am her pet her lover

And I don't worry about the others.

Yesterday I gave the Grand Cherokee back to Mara even though she does not have a license or insurance yet and keeps the ten thousand I gave her in a shoe box for fear of creditors.

Last night after I made love to her petite toes with my tongue, Mistress had me dress like a whore in red nightie, blond wig, red lipstick and high heels. She put on over her jeans a strap on and made me get to my knees and suck until she began to fuck me in the mouth. After awhile she made me lay on the bed, head over the edge so she could fuck my mouth while seeing my face and eyes. Then she had me get on the bed and show her my pussy. She started gently but before long she fucked me with vigor and I knew I was her slut and slave and lover forever.

Now I sit in my chair typing wearing red panties and ringed collar knowing I cannot play with my cock without permission. Sitting on the table are weighted nipple clamps that will make me reaffirm my loyalty and love for Mistress. For she loves slaves that take pain for her. She hit me hard with her hard leather triangular strap as she fucked me.

Oh god. I must get on my hands and knees and worship Mistress even in her absence. If I come on the floor I must lick it up. I must wait for permission and workout hard for her. For from the workouts followed by sleep comes vibrancy.

8:30 a.m. I did not run this morning. Instead I read and dozed in bed and now I am doing floor exercises and weights.

Today I must finish the business plan as soon as possible. Perhaps I will work from home this morning. I finally figured out how to get my messages off the phone after it has been screwed up for so long.

My home. Last night Mistress told me that she thought we should get a bed for the loft and I said I had a bed. She said you have a mattress—she thinks of beds as wood and headboards and such stuff. We agreed that she would not redo the bed until we moved in together. Soon! I want that to happen sooner rather than later. I want to live with Mara my Mistress even if it is in a cage under the bed.

She told me she has had a life-long dream of having her own dungeon. Right now she has her whips and paddles and collars and leashes and nipple clamps hanging on the walls in my back room.

Sometimes I wonder how I am so lucky to have a beautiful goddess as my Mistress and future wife. I hope this is not a dream that will come crashing down around me so that I become a vagabond on the streets with only stories to tell.

Fate teases the greedy.

Arrive late to the party

And discover it is not for you.

But I awake

From my nightmare to a kiss

Of my Mistress on my

Trembling lips.

This is Tuesday. The last week before I turn fifty. Cheryl already had an ice cream cake for the March and April birthdays.

I have known two people who had birthdays on April 3. My college roommate who was two years older and a woman poet who is several years younger. My college roommate ran the student film program for the college I attended. I met the woman poet at the same place I met Mara, a bar for people with fetishes. Both of them worked there only short intervals and quit.

Friends. I have many friends, but would I have friends if this journal were published? Would I have a job? Interesting thought. If I came out as the BDSM slave of Mistress Mara would my coworkers shun me?

Today I must clean up many small items: letters and responses to resumes and such stuff. I must prepare for arguments in the Court of Appeals. Twenty-three pushups and it elevated my heart rate to 115.

I fight a huge conflict of wanting to work here at home and the need to go into the office to show my co-workers I am there working even though I will get less done.

I only have today left. Consider that possibility. So spend each moment as if you only have this day left. Live it fully doing what I do with the presence of making each letter, each phrase, written or spoke with thought and depth.

In the past few weeks I have found a best friend in Trevor Pale. Beyond that I love Mistress and have discovered the joy of touching her and talking to her. She says she enjoys being with me and loves me. Let myself enjoy this day in that realization.

Go. Get ready and get to the office! I have little hope for income this month but see what you can do. Relax and stay in the moment! Each moment of life deserves my attention. Stress kills the possibilities, let the stress go. Perhaps I will compose my daily work in this journal, at least some of it because if I do it with intensity and passion, it too will have a beauty. Go.

Fifty arrives. I shall not ever claim conventionality. Unique. As Tom Robbins said in a paragraph: "unique" means one-of-a-kind and should not be used as a generic descriptor.

I must make my greatest weaknesses my greatest strengths. I have been saying that to myself for days, now I must make it happen!!!! Thank god I am writing again. I have not played a game of online scrabble in days nor have I spent time online looking at profiles or cams. I have thrust myself back into the world with the help of my friends. My trainer is a sought after model. Trevor my collaborator and soon-to-be partner. Each has taken a role and Mistress with her love and support.

And this journal, written mostly on Sajina my laptop computer has a healing effect by itself. Writing brings focus on the moment.

11AM. Mara called me and we discussed my concerns. She told me not to worry that she loved me very much and that her phone had died and she could not find the charger. I love her unconditionally and I do not question her I just worry about her. She laughed and said, "If something happens you will be the first to know." She also told me to bill hours today which I will do.

She is flying to Las Vegas on Thursday morning and comes back Sunday or Monday. She said she hopes to earn some money while she is there. The photo shoot is on Friday all day. What she does while she is there. I appreciate that she is independent. Enough that she loves me and that is all.

Chapter Nine
March 29, 2006 Wed.

(Writing from Stephan's notebook written at The Common Grounds where he ate lunch)

I was at the office at 7:30 a.m. this morning and met with an accountant and an associate of his about the theater. They are going to help me get Blues House up and running.

I have to get prepared for the Court of Appeals. I am going to spend hours in preparation. Money doesn't matter now. The key is making Blues House work correctly.

I see Kiowa, the German Shepard, running to get her ball and bringing it back to me to throw again.

"Call me at anytime to ask." Conversation from the next table. Two women talking about business. Last night….

Cool. You are firing finery finally falling through the fissures.

Chapter Ten
March 30, 2006

1:30PM. I plan to go home to work on preparation for arguments. That way I can write as well.

7:00PM. I did not go home and now I am back at the office. Rachel stopped by and we ate at Forest Room 5. She has given up trying to shake my love for Mara and we are just friends that talk. Mara sent me a text message from Las Vegas saying that she got there and that she loved me.

I haven't worked hard in three days or at least I have not done a walk run in three days and I have gained back the weight I lost. Crazy. I am stressed. Tomorrow I must work on Court of Appeals arguments all day long. My knee hurts. I did not sleep last night because I ate too much fried chicken. I have failed to get much done today except reconnect with people. One of them is interested in investing in the theater space.

Chapter Eleven
April 1, 2006, 1:55 A.M.

I failed to write yesterday and I failed to work on the appeal argument that is to occur on my birthday. However, yesterday may have been the day that changed my life for good. In some ways it was a perfect day. At 6 am in the morning I walked and ran around Cheesman Park. What can I remember now? Lately, I have thought that soon I would break through my workout barriers and run the entire distance. I didn't do that. I walked up the hill on 9th Avenue and stopped to stretch my calves using a tree to lean against like one side of a triangle. I ran for maybe three minutes on the way to the park and then decided to walk when I started breathing heavily. Although it was light no one was sitting outside at Diedrich's Coffee on 9th and Downing by the King Sooper's that people call the Queen Sooper's because there are so many of the gay community that shop there. If I ever feel the need to exhibit my body (if I get in shape) I merely need to walk or run through the sidewalk seating at the coffee shop. Even in my present weight lifter physique I get some looks.

When I reached the park and turned onto the dirt track I still walked a few yards. I remember thinking that if I ran all the way around the park that I would have to run those few walked yards to make the full lap. It did not matter because I only ran to the southeast corner of the park and then stopped to walk. In the chill air I wore sweatpants and a sweatshirt and walking ahead of me was an old man in shorts and a t-shirt walking with a gait that seemed like he would try but fail to break into a run every fourth stride.

I break my chronology for a moment to recognize that my writing has transformed, at least for the moment, into a detailed examination of the observed.

8 a.m. My focus on writing failed when the computer crashed the program and I lost a full paragraph. I ended up going to bed then waking sexually aroused wanting to have someone come over and play but I didn't because I am owned by Mistress. What I do sexually is totally her call. So instead I cross dressed in a black skirt white shirt, blond wig, eye liner, red lipstick and white knee high and turned on the cam and performed for various voyeurs. I got very high ratings. Mistress has channeled my sexuality and I avoided spending money on an escort and avoided hooking up with some unknown person. I watched a transsexual sex movie that I have and came once and then an hour or two later came again. Maybe it is the vitamins I have been taking. Maybe Mara stimulates me even when she is not here. That is a true statement. I hope she does well in Vegas and has a portfolio to show for it. I was disappointed that I paid for Mark the photographer to come out here at Mara's insistence then she decided to go back to Vegas for the photos and spent another two or three thousand dollars. Mara spends money like she was drinking water. She spends thousands in a few days. She told me the ten thousand I gave her she would parley into fifty thousand. We shall see. Now she has the truck and ten thousand and a credit card with a limit of 2500 that she maxed out in a few days. I paid it down a thousand. I love her but financially she kills me.

Then I read more of Rita's book. It is very good. Not great, but it holds my attention.

Back to yesterday. When I passed the old man with walk-run gait I looked at him and saw his sunken cheeks and big lips of old age. When I said hello he clearly heard me—totally cognitive and said hello to me. When I got most of the way around Cheesman three women who had been ahead of me stopped and hugged the bigger one who left the park. They ran past me. There were two tall blond Amazon women runners who were talking and talking and met me twice and never saw me.

Oh, and on the way to the park I said hello to a woman with two dogs going two different directions. On my hello she looked at me and said hi. For some reason it reminded me of New Orleans when I was 18 and said hello to a woman on Bourbon Street. I thought that the woman I said hi to in 1978 would be old now, just the age of the woman with the dogs. I almost cried.

Then the day started in earnest. I went to a coffee shop for my weekly meeting with Trevor. I arrived on time at 7:30 AM and guy at the counter took my order and said, "I didn't think you got up so early."

The owner of the coffee shop next door to the theater said he is more excited about us finishing the theater and getting started than we are. Not possible but he is very into our project.

Now I going to go running and come back and finish my writing and spend the rest of the day preparing for the oral arguments. Trevor had written some amazing stuff for the web site for Blues House. I met with the retailers in the building with the theater and we discussed sending letter of intent to the landlord for the purchase of the properties. We agreed to meet at 1:30 pm at coffee shop and finish the letter. I went back to the office and worked on various things but finished the letter of intent.

So we start down the road. I have new partners in a new world. Then I went and got my driver's license. I stood in line for 40 minutes and when I dropped the paper to the ground I had difficulty bending to pick it up. Parkinson's disease sucks. When everyone had left the office I stopped in Shane's office and talked to him about the firm and what I have been doing. He said we have to use the theater to market the firm and I said the firm would have to put some money into it and he said of course. Good. A reaction I did not expect. I told him he should watch Boston Legal and see the scenes between the senior partners at the end of the show. He said he had his baseball glove in the car and I have mine in my office so we can go out and throw someday when we have a little time. We connected for a few moments which was very good.

Then I got a call from Rachel who asked if she could get another loan of $1500. She is desperate, trying to find a job but too proud to take on roommates or take a 12 dollar an hour job. I told her that if she came over last night and picked up the check I would loan her the money. She offered to cook dinner and we talked in my newly rearranged living room which is rearranged on angles and she was amazed at how attractive it is with the various sitting areas and the paint. I set it up for comfort and communication. Entertaining guests delights me now. We watched Secretary the movie about BDSM until it got to the heavier BDSM part.

She does not fully understand how happy I am as the slave of Mistress Mara, my fiancée and future wife.

So yesterday I made the offer on behalf of the retailers to purchase the retail space and my entire work life is changing. If I can make this project happen, I will change my entire style of working and living. I intend to work from home and to spend incredible hours at the theater. I will coordinate with the other retailers and the entire project should skyrocket. Theater on the rail. The Blues House Theater has captured the imaginations of many.

11:46 a. m. I walked and ran around Cheesman. Much more walking than running-I would be happy with my life if I were 180 and running consistently. I got my driver's license yesterday and had to say my weight was 240 lbs.

1:00 PM. I just woke from a nap in the recliner. Weight 239, 60 pounds must come off as soon as possible! Now focus on prepping for court. Fifty shall be synonymous with change. Mapping each day as if there were a treasure waiting for me. Like the girl on a bike with a wide grin.

Or Mistress's message to me saying that the photo shoot went well. I must lose weight every day. No choice. Do it!

Chapter Twelve
April 2, 2006.

9:52 pm. I am at home dictating to the computer, dictating to Sajina on Dragon Speak. I spent much of this day before my birthday preparing for Oral arguments in the Court of Appeals. I have been happy and sad today. I was sad because I discovered that Mara had booked her flight back from Las Vegas late tomorrow night so she would miss my birthday. I don't know that she did so that she would miss my birthday but the effect was the same. I pled with her to come home early and she did agree to do that but she had me send $600 by Western Union to her. Recently I gave her $10,000 and my vehicle the Jeep Cherokee. She told me she was going to take the $10,000 and make 50,000. I doubted her statement and now I doubted it even more. She spends money like it was tap water.

Is very important to me that she comes back to Denver to celebrate my 50th birthday and have dinner with myself, Gray Mackey and his girlfriend Natalia. She is young like Mara. When I talked to Mara on the phone she kept talking about how she had wanted to go shopping and spent about thousand dollars. He also sound of said that she had to come back because she was going to be looking for an agent in Las Vegas. So I told her we would go back in a few weeks. I need to schedule Mother and Father coming here and the trip to Washington DC.

I fell asleep dictating. The dictation is good because it makes me form my words carefully.

Date	Running Description/location	Total workout tin

Thur 3/23/06	2min/3min/1minu- CH park	One hour
Saturday 3/25/06	2 laps CH park	One hour +
Sunday 3/26/06	Focused on Speed - CH park	One hour
Monday 3/27/06	3 - 3-min. intervals – fluid running 1 lap CH park	One hour
Wed 3/29/06	20 min floor and stationary bike	20 min
Friday 3/31/06	1 lap CH park 3-3 min intervals	One hour.
Saturday 4/1/06	1 lap CH park 4-2 min intervals	One hour
Sunday 4/2/06	1 lap CH park 5-2 min intervals	One hour

So I start typing manually. I need to work on legal stuff but I believe I should sleep now and wake early to do that.

Thoughts: work ethic. Tough as nails. Run in the morning as well as prep.

I received a message from Rita saying Happy Birthday to me as a friend and her mentor. Her book made me laugh out loud tonight. Then I prepared to argue.

On my run tonight I started examining the oral arguments from an imaging point of view. I have to do more of that when I wake.

So I will wake fifty and my issues have not resolved yet. Tomorrow will be interesting.

Chapter Thirteen
April 3 2006 4:30AM

So I am now fifty years old. A new decade of my life. Assessment, I love where I live. I have a positive net worth. I am working on the biggest personal project of my lifetime, no actually the two biggest projects of my lifetime, no actually the five biggest projects of my lifetime. Each of them is a lifetime endeavors.

1. My relationship with Mara who I love more and more each day;
2. Putting my body back to marathon shape for the rest of my life.
3. Holding together a law firm with my old classmate, Shane Heitman and two amazing youngsters and an aging singer-actress. I have to write more about them later.
4. Building a theater in the middle of the city.
5. Writing creatively and publishing. This is multiple projects including this one which I doubt I will have guts enough to publish while I am alive.

I weigh 240, have a Mistress and a model as a girlfriend, have a super-model as a trainer, have run three days in a row and plan to do so this morning.

Damn I am burning the pork chops I put on the stove!!!

They were ok I had the stove turned low. I am cooking a package that had been sitting in the fridge and mixing with rice for a nutritious meal that I can put in a plastic container.

I need better focus and discipline and a tough work ethic. If I can get my body in shape that it can run marathons I will be able to achieve every one of my goals easier.

Now prepare for oral arguments and run. First I will read some key cases.

6:26 a.m. I found the key cases and read them. Then I composed a message to Mara and sent by email.

Mistress

I love you very much and I want you to know you are the number one priority in my life for the rest of my life. Without you the color would go out of my days. I would lose the edge of creativity that has returned to my writing. I would have no reason of accomplishing the other things in my life that I dedicate to you. I promise to be honest and tell you everything no matter what I think or do because you are my lover, my confidant, my best friend and my Mistress.

As I write and think about our relationship, I understand that it is extraordinary to find someone like you who understands me and desires what I desire not just sexually but in life generally, creativity, family, entrepreneurship, and you do.

This morning very early I started working on preparing for my oral arguments today but I stopped to write you this affirmation of my love and my intent to be there for you no matter what. I deeply appreciate you coming back for my birthday and I know how important it is to you to find an agent. Sometimes I worry about all the money spent but quite frankly money is money and money is nothing. What is important in life is our relationships with people and with our mate most of all. Our relationship has so many layers and it is deepening and getting stronger every day. I heard disappointment in your voice at not being able to look for an agent and it is that disappointment that makes me love you more because you are coming back to see me when I most need you.

Your Slave lover and friend

Stephan

6:37PM. Mara did not show up for dinner. She did not send me a message back and I did not hear from her until mid-afternoon when she was going to the airport. She did not say what she did last night or today and told me at 4pm that the airlines had told her they were booked. Frankly I do not believe her otherwise she would have called me back this morning. Then there was a little fiasco of getting 600 through Western Union that she had me send. Now I am just going to see what happens. I am very disappointed she did not figure out how to get back for my birthday and her total absorption in herself so that she just plain forgot my birthday and scheduled her flight so she would not get back makes me think about my decisions and devotion. Does she care? Does she love me? Or is it just money for her? Am I just a source of money and vehicle and does she just endure me so that she has money? This is very nearly the same as Christmas. I bought her an expensive coat at her insistence and then she did not even buy me a present. Now I bought her a portfolio and she cannot even get back for my fiftieth birthday. I guess I will go have dinner with Gray and Natalia and worry about this later.

Chapter Fourteen
April 4, 2006.

Ironically, Mara called last night after I returned from dinner and she was excited. She had gone into a Christian Dior store and saw three things that she loved: a dress for $2800, a pair of shoes and a purse for $2000 and she called me to have me sent her two thousand dollars by Western Union after she had just received $600 from me by Western Union that I had sent the night before. She was very excited about the purse and shoes and she told me she would pay back the $2000 but we both know better.

However, I am her bitch and ultimately whatever she tells me to do I will do because I love her beyond belief. If someone is reading this my actions are probably beyond their belief too. I guess you could put it this way, love is when you send $2000 to your lover who has missed being with you on your 50th birthday at 10 p.m. at night after getting back from a dinner which she missed so she can buy a purse and shoes in Las Vegas just before she flies home. Either it is love or I'm incredibly stupid. Probably both, because they are not mutually exclusive. Only time will give me the answers to the question of whether my love was foolish or fantastic. I can say I am not stupid because I am following the more important path of love. Money is meaningless for me now or at least it should be. After all she may be supporting me soon.

The fire alarm went off actually and metaphorically. I must go run and stay on track today. I can write later of cleaning out the closet and how it is so analogous to writing this piece. Writing is paramount but getting my body in shape is even more important. Conditioning begets creativity. Today will be the fifth day in a row to do the Cheesman route. I slept little last night so it will be interesting to see how I do.

Chapter Fifteen
April 5, 2006

12:30 a.m.

I remember my father reading late into the night. He would sit with his feet up smoking a pipe at his place by the kitchen table next to the back door which was the most used door. When he wasn't smoking the pipe he would bang it on a pipe stand made of cast-iron. Certain noises bring back my father's image to me, the banging of a pipe and the tapping of glass on the table. Stacks of books also remind me of him.

Collections of glass figures remind me of my mother. A year or so ago I had her conduct a tour of the house and her collections and I videotaped it. I should find that videotape and treasure it.

Tonight Rachel invited me over to her house after class, my business planning class, and I stopped in and watch the show Boston Legal which has made me cry on several occasions due to the relationship between the characters played by James Spader and William Shatner.

After the show Rachel gave me a birthday card and flowers and presents. The presents were candles, wine glasses and wine and a perfect present, a set of ink pens, the kind you dip in ink. I should know the word for the pens but at this time of night I don't.

For some reason it is very difficult to dictate tonight. Perhaps I need to dictate faster and with more complexity for Dragon Speak to work. I spoke briefly to Mara today and discovered that she just flew into Denver and that she had spent the night in Las Vegas and had bought the shoes and purse for which I sent to her $2000 on my birthday. Then she stayed at another hotel that a client of hers got her and conducted an hour long session for him. Now I just wait to see whether she has any thought to treat me nicely or whether I'm just a source of money for her. Days like today make me think I'm just a source of money for her. When she gets on her feet financially will she pay my back as she said? Or is she just going to keep getting more and more money from me? When I gave her the $$10,000 in cash she told me she would turn it into $50,000 and put it back into the theater. I guess this journal shall tell the tale of whether I am stupid or rightfully in love with Mara who loves me as much as she says. She has yet to have me over to the house for which I paid rent all three months if you count the $10,000 which she will use for this month's rent. She ran up the credit card that I gave her to the maximum $2500 within a few days after she got the card. I even paid it down another thousand. I paid the photographer 1800 for her portfolio and to come to Denver to shoot. He was going to reimburse part of that? Am I just a source of money? She has yet to stay with me for one night and we are engaged. Am I a fool or does she truly love me? Now I am not sure.

I must sleep so I can run for the sixth day in a row.

8am. I walked and ran for the sixth straight day. Now I sit here wearing my collar, nipple clamps and cockstrap and I realize that Mistress owns me from my soul out. I love her and whether I am a fool or not doesn't matter since she owns me and everything I have. Just accept the fact and all will turn out well.

Vitamins focus and shower.

Chapter Sixteen
Saturday April 8, 2006

4am on a Saturday morning. I slept a little and ended up watching a Goldie Hawn and Steve Martin movie that made me cry. He won her by telling stories as she was about to leave on the bus. I don't know the name of the movie, but I am going to look up the movie on Amazon and buy it.

This morning will be the 9th day in a row of walking/running in the morning. If I can start controlling my late night eating I will start dropping weight.

7:30am. This has been an exhausting night. I ordered the movie Housesitters with Steve Martin and Goldie Hawn which is the one I watched. Actually I only saw about half of it and I look forward to getting the movie. I also ordered Dirty Rotten Scoundrels and a nonfiction book.

Mara was supposed to come by last night, but did not – I have not seen her since at least the day before she left for Las Vegas, the trip that cost me at least 5000 dollars. I hope the pictures came out well. It sounds as if Mara is about out of money thus effectively spending 17,500 dollars in about 30 days. 10,000 cash, 2,500 on the credit card, 1800 to the photographer, 650 western union and 2,200 western union for the purse and shoes. This is ridiculous. I have spent well over 100,000 on Mara since July of last year. Let alone in essence giving her the truck. She has to pay for herself. I have to pay taxes that are probably due. This is crazy crazy crazy. I should end this relationship, but I cannot, I love her. She doesn't show up or do things with me, she spends my money and she tells me that she loves me and is going to marry me and we are going to live together. Am I stupid or does she love me. She missed my fiftieth birthday and didn't even see me in the week afterwards. Am I absolutely off my rocker?

Then I think about my ex-girlfriend Rachel who recently asked for another 1500 dollars. She wrote in her journal about me, "I just can't believe me of all people, got suckered by such a drone." Later she wrote,

> Stephan decided finally to bless us with his presence here at the house. I had finally good enough about the situation to start reorganizing the place and making it look even cleaner and more comfortable. Needless to say I was uncomfortable with the idea of this abomination coming back to turn it into a pig sty. Even if he knew what clean and orderly was, I still don't want to have to share the company with a disillusioned zombie again. MAN! I can't believe I put up with that crap for long!! And he STILL has no idea how it has been. As a matter of fact, I'll bet he is still telling people that we are not together because I hate the theatre and we have different interests. What a moron. I wonder if he'll ever realize it is because he is a highly self-absorbed maniac lost in space.

She went on and on. It is ironic that now she disses Mara and gets me birthday presents and calls me her best friend. Perhaps I am, but the bottom line is I am the same person.

Last week the law firm was falling apart.

11pm on Saturday night.

I still haven't seen Mara because she and a new girl she "hired" are working at my loft doing domination. I talked to her a few moments ago and told her I wanted to book a session and she laughed and said, "You are funny." Earlier she had said they might work until 4am. I said, "Money in the door." It was awful though hearing a man's voice in the background in my loft while I am at work.

However, I did some essential research on the proposed new case involving a cosmetic company. It is for trademark infringement and involves a substitute for the stuff that Mara puts in her lips.

I keep intending to write about last week after the oral arguments. At the rate I am going to fall asleep at my computer. It was something to consider

This os wjatt jpta'jiiippppppppthatsaaaaaaaaaaaaaaaaaaaaaaaaaaaaaaaaaaaaaaa aaaaaaaaaaaaaaaaaaaaaaaaaaaaaaaaaaaaaaaaaaaaaaaaaaaaaaaaaaaa aaaaaaaaaaaaaaaaaaaaaaaaaaaaaaaaaaaaaaaaaaaaaaaaaaaaaaaaaaaa aaaaaaaaaaaaaaaaaaaaaaaaaaaaaaaaaaaaaaaaaaaaaaaaaaaaaaaaaaaa aaaaaaaaaaaaaaaaaaaaaaaaaaaaaaaaaaaaaaaaaaaaaaaaaaaaaaaaaaaa aaaddddddddddddddddddddddddddddddddddddddddddddddddddd dddddddddddddddddddddddddddddddddddddddddddddddddddddddd dddddddssssssssssss

No corrections, although I am exhausted.

Last week Cheryl almost quit due to the fact that Shane ssssssssssssssssssssssssssssssssssssssssssssssssssssssssssssssssss ssssssssssssssssssssssssss stresses her out when we work together. I would sleep in Sam's chair but Janice is here working on a case. I have to bag it now. The bright points were a series of new clients from h343 o4 5hi\34l.wwwwwwwwwwwwwwwwwwwwwwwwwwqqqqqqqqqqq qqqqqqqqqqqqqqqqqqqqqqqqqqqqqqqqqq'''''''''''''''''''''''''''''' ''.

I am so tired I cannot competently put words on paper. The Parkisinion nnnnnnnnnnnnnnnnnnnnnnnnnnnnnnnnn

Chapter Seventeen
April 9, 2006

Sunday morning at exactly 10 a.m.

Mara! Life amazes. Yesterday started innocuously and predictably. The Pilipino woman who cleans my loft was late. I tried to open a bank account in the morning and forgot to bring the tax identification number.

12:44 am on April 10, 2006. I am continuing Chapter Seventeen as the story of this weekend because I did not get to write it down yesterday. Yesterday flowed easily but Saturday reversed my life direction at least twice. Mara's can bend me with her will as if I were a molten piece of steel. Her voice heats me like the licking flames of the torch.

I am molten metal

Heated by the licking flames

Of your voice.

For you to shape

With your breath

With your mind

And with your soul.

Magma as I am

Longing for cool

Sizzling touch

Of your fingers

And soft humm

Of a voice that torched me

And now cools my fiery existence

Into a mirrored finish

Displaying the image

I adore.

You.

 You have come for me

My angel from heaven and hell

And gladly

I melt my soul into yours.

6:05 am. I just sent the poem I wrote earlier this morning to Mara. For my birthday she gave me a framed picture of her in an angel outfit with wings. When I walked home from the Hyatt where I stayed on Saturday night or rather Sunday morning, I saw that picture and a hand-written note.

April 11, 2006. 2:05 am.

    I am sitting upstairs at the computer named Gandalf that provides a clear view of the mountains to the West when the shade is open. I woke after 3 hours of sleep and poured myself an orange juice laced with Magnesium to relax my muscles.

    My loft has become Mara's place of work and Alice has become a friend. This past Saturday morning, April 9, 2006, I had no clue that Alice was in town or that she helping Mara. Last night I pulled my jeep up beside my Cherokee which Alice had parked in the North American Title parking lot below and to the east of my loft. I offered Alice dry roasted peanuts which she declined.

I am starting to tire and soon I must go back to sleep but I need to capture images of the past few days before they disappear into the mist of time. Camus observed that man forgets even the good he has done. Yesterday I met with a well-known playwright and director and told him our vision of the Blues House theater. Not only is he in, he said our vision is what art is about. He will help in any way he can. I believe I will ask him to join the board of directors. We are idealists who, as Trevor, the black man with dreads, who grew up in Kansas, said, "still believe in Dorothy and the yellow-brick road."

Mara called me Saturday night while I sat on the wall overlooking Cherry Creek river and talked to me and told me she loved me and was going to marry me and told me to give Alice a chance. I had lost my cool and become very angry when I discovered Alice sitting in the Cherokee outside the lofts. I thought she had left Mara's life forever. She has made love to Mara, more than I have and I am engaged to Mara. The last I heard of Alice was when I got a criminal defense lawyer to help Mara when Alice was arrested for trying to cash what was said to be forged money orders. Alice did not know that and was not responsible for the forgery but her name caused me angst.

On Sunday night I dreamed I died. I felt that I was in a vortex and my mind was shutting off. I recognized death and accepted death and then woke up. Now I shall go to sleep and then come back to write more.

For whom do I write this journal? For Mara my lover and future wife who is so strong despite her youth. To discover how the mysteries of life unfolded to me. For others so they can learn to understand themselves. For myself to discover the world I live in. It is 3:25 am and I have still not drawn the image of Alice and myself driving around town at 3am on Saturday night looking for a coffee shop that wasn't crowded. We met at the Colorado Café which was mobbed and went by Pete's kitchen which was equally mobbed. I showed her where the theater would be. She asked, "why would you put the theater in the 'hood." I have to use that, "Theater in the 'hood."

Then we drove Colfax and while Alice answered calls for Mara who was working at the loft doing domination sessions, we discussed my story ideas for a My Fair Lady hip hop parody and for the musical Colfax. Alice could help me with both because she is an "industry-lady" as Mara says and writes rap, hip-hop and poetry.

I still had not seen Mara since a day before she left for Las Vegas for the photo shoot and ended up staying four days. Mara had Alice drop me off at the Hyatt where I stayed the rest of the night and watched "Capote" before walking home on Sunday morning. Now it is 3:37 am and I must sleep. I will email this to myself so I can access it at the office.

6:34 a. m. So finally I slept hard and now I will go run/ walk for the twelfth straight day. Perhaps today I will run the park and stop for coffee.

Chapter Eighteen
April 12, 2006

Wed. 12:30 pm. I was the first person in the office again today. I got here at 7:50 am and no one else showed up until 8:30am. Yesterday, I did not run until nighttime, but I did run. I ran half of Cheesman, the uphill half. However, I did not finish the lap so I did not stop for the celebratory coffee. Soon I hope. If I run tonight it will be thirteen days in a row. The weight is starting to decrease.

Chapter Nineteen
Saturday April 15, 2006

6:00 a.m. I did not run on Wednesday night. Days are starting to blur again and I need to catch myself and write. I do not have a cord for Sajina which is the computer I am using to write at this moment. There are a few minutes left on the battery and I wonder if I should switch computers.

Last night I think I was schizophrenic if I know what that means. I love Mara and more and more to remind me of characters played by Goldie Hawn. In fact, I'm beginning to wonder if Mara might not be a wonderful actress.

Last night I was schizophrenic if that means being to separate individuals on the same evening. First of all we were scheduled to have dinner with Gray Mackey and his girlfriend Natalia from Romania. We were scheduled at 7 PM at PF Changs in the Park Meadows Shopping Center. I arrived before 7 PM and talked to Mara who told me she was a few minutes away. I waited. At a little after seven Gray Mackey and Natalia arrived. They got a buzzer that would let us know when the table is ready. We waited. I spoke to Mara who told me she was a few minutes away still. At about 15 after seven I told them to go inside and get the table when the buzzer rang. I waited. Finally at 7:20 p.m. I called Mara again and she said she was a few minutes away so I should go in and sit down. I did. We waited for Mara. Finally at 745 I called her again and she told me that she taken the wrong Highway and had to circle back. Finally she arrived about one hour late.

So in early January, January 14 to be precise I went to a play at the Mercury Café. Gray and Natalia were there and I came and Mara did not arrive. I think that she was sick that night. Then on April 3

Gray and Natalia were scheduled to have dinner with Mara and myself or my 50th birthday. Mara did not make it back from Las Vegas and I ate dinner with them on my 50th birthday and ended up sending $2000 by Western Union so that Mara could buy a pair of shoes and a purse. She missed her plane and did not get back until Tuesday. Eventually several days later she gave me a picture of herself in a frame for my 50th birthday along with a note. However, the first time I saw her after April 3 was at a Target store in Aurora where she had me meet her and I bought $500 worth of stuff for her business being done in the loft.

I have yet to be invited to the house I'm paying for on South Andes Way. Mara does not think of my feelings much or so it seems to me. Still, I love her dearly. The dinner was extraordinary but probably more extraordinary from Gray and Natalia's point of view than mine. But more about the dinner later now I have to go run. The battery is running down and I need to get the charger for this computer. There's much to be written about including throwing a baseball at lunch with my law partner. However, the most interesting story to write was the story Mara told to Gray and Natalia because it was so shocking to them.

So now I go run and see if I can justify buying coffee to celebrate a full lap around Cheesman Park.

3:00 p.m. Mara left a note with her picture downstairs. It said:

Stephan

"Happy Birthday. I love you so much and I miss you like crazy. Be secure in the fact that I want you and that we will be married. Soon our wedding pix will be in these frames. Love you and happy birthday."

Mara

So no matter what happens we will work through it.

3:55 p.m.   So one week ago I went through a rollercoaster Saturday in which I was ready for a short while to leave Mara and ended up finding out that Alice, a black girl from Sacramento, California was actually quite cool. I was upset with Mara because I discovered that Alice had come back into her life before she told me and I knew Alice as her former lover. Mara assured me she had told Alice we were getting married and that Alice was invited to the wedding. Last Saturday, after Mara put us together, Alice and I drove around and we talked about writing, creativity and the theater. We agreed to go to spoken word events together.

I am tired. A short nap is in order. Soon I have to work.

7:24 p. m. I had a long telephone conversation with Mara and have eaten a supper of rice and beans. During my conversation with Mara, with her instigation and encouragement, I fucked myself with a dildo stuck to the wall. It was the dildo she uses in her strap on to fuck me. She enjoyed it as much as I. She and I share our kinkiness and a love for our odd mistress slave sexual relationship, although our full relationship is far more complex.

Every downturn in our relationship ultimately seems to strengthen the relationship. I need her desperately. She is my Mistress and my future wife and my friend.

Chapter Twenty
April 16, 2006

5:30 a. m. Easter Sunday. This is day fourteen of my fiftieth year. Is this my last day of life? I overate yesterday and I weighed 240 after being 235. I should run again this morning but instead I will write and go in and do the work I should have done yesterday. If I haven't killed or maimed myself by the kinkiness I need to focus on getting the brief done that is due later this week.

I am almost out of money. If Jimmy Dice had not agreed to lend me 50,000 dollars I would be panicked.

How life changes. On December 31, 2000 I angrily wrote:

> The year 2000 comes to a close. I've learned much including in the past few days. Jimmy Dice went berserk angry on the telephone with me yesterday—he was screaming and I told him to get control and call me back. He said, "You call yourself a lawyer." He didn't apologize when he called me back. So I spent one half million dollars of my time for an unintelligent (basically dumb) salesman who can't control his temper. He is a "client" not a friend. When these cases are done, I'm done with him.

Well, I had no clue what the future would bring and how smart Jimmy really was even though at the time he yelled at me he was probably drunk. He changed his life; we changed our lives. Now he saves me by telling me that I can borrow $50,000 at the drop of a hat.

On January 1, 2001 I wrote about having a shaky scribbling hand and I wrote that walks are good for creativity. I wrote about creativity then and on January 7, 2001 I removed my body hair for the first time. Rachel told me for the first time she did not like body hair and called me a pervert for wanting to take nude pictures of her. Amusing. Wednesday she left a message on my phone that I looked great. How times change. It is now 6 a.m. on Sunday morning April 16, 2006. Soon I have to go to the office.

Mara and I talked several times on the telephone yesterday.

7:30 a.m. I slept some more and I am starting to feel better.

8:19 I am eating a warmed over crock pot concoction of roast beef, potatoes and red peppers that I had saved in the refrigerator. How can I gain pounds in a day? I did. I wanted to weigh in below 230 and instead I am 240. Yesterday I did two laps around Cheesman. What is the problem and how do I conquer the desire to eat? Discipline. Focus. I write words on the page now instead of putting them on the scrabble board. I must discipline myself in all aspects of life.

Rachel, my ex-girlfriend asked me for $1500 last month and I gave it to her. She is doing the graphic design for the theater. But isn't it interesting to consider that a few years ago when I was in the depths of depression and problems I was in her words "too fucked up to wait for." I am still a fat man trying to avoid the coffin (a clay sculpture of mine) but I am making the effort and for the first time in my life I truly am in love. Mara. Mara. A friend said I should write Mara's story and Alice said, "Mara is a trip, in a good way."

Fifty and Change. The quarters click in my pocket against the nickels and dimes.

I saw a postcard with an actor named Anthony advertising Death of a Salesman at the Fox. He has been back in town but has not called. I bailed him out of a financial issue with a credit card—essentially gave him a thousand or two dollars. However, why would he call? I have not tried calling him while he was in L.A. and the good thing is that he is still acting, still practicing his art. The day I weigh in at 180 which better be sooner rather than later, I am going to sign up for the first audition I can find.

I believe Mara has the opportunity to become a world famous actress. She has the Goldie Hawn style and most of all the Goldie Hawn confidence. Perhaps I should say the Mistress Mara confidence. Yes Mara is a trip!! And I am on that trip. What roads shall we travel? Many roads very fast. Hold on!!!!

9:00 P.M. A very good day. I worked eight hours on the brief. I worked with Janice I realized how much she supports me. The Parkinson's strikes me at times and puts me in la la land. Janice helps me get through those times. I got to the office at ten a.m. and worked until 5:00 p.m. Really the only time I was not working I spent talking to Greg about the theater. Greg has liver cancer and is on chemotherapy. I told him today what an example he is to me. His love of the theater and his dedication to the Blues House project makes me realize how lucky I am to have him blessing this theater. His spirit will infuse the Blues House forever.

I suppose my life has changed because after dinner at PF Changs, where Mara told all, Gray and Natalia now know Mara and me more intimately than any of my other friends. I hope Natalia and Mara become close friends, shopping buddies and I hope Gray is intrigued, not put off.

When Natalia and Gray said they were getting married this summer, Mara said, "Maybe we can make it a double wedding."

I want to marry Mara but I want to be 180 pounds when I do it. Even 190 would work but that is fifty or sixty pounds lighter than I am right now. Enough of this obsession with weight. Now I shall take care of the weight and at the same time write of new ideas.

Poetry, plays and essays written in every spare moment.

Ten years ago, give or take a few months, I was in Guilford, England staying at a client's home in Surrey. I wrote:

> Mon. 1-15-96. 7 Am. In Denver it's about midnight. Here I'm making coffee and preparing to run. This notebook was the best I could find in Guilford with a minimum of looking after I realized I was running out of paper.

(The notebook is green with a big "RECYCLE" on the front)

I wrote on:

> Plato—"The unexamined life is not worth living." When you truly see, the colors are more intense.

Not only did I scribble words, I sketched pictures: a cover for my book Knights of the Nebraska Round Table; sketches of helmets for knights; a blanketed beggar sitting cross-legged at the bottom of the stairs in the underground. Then I wrote a poem:

I tell you my friend if you are to live,
You must see.

Yet,
You say
I have no eyes
And I tell you can see without eyes
For
If I had no eyes I'd see through my ears
And my fingers and tongue.
You say to me
I can't hear
And I ask
How do you communicate with me
And I hear
"I don't know"
From you.
"Yesterday," I say,
I smelled decaying leaves
Along the roadside
And burnt wood
Near a cottage.
You are silent now
And refuse to try
So I must walk on
My sympathy only
For those who seek life
And fail,
Dropping from the rocks they climb,
Not for those
Who seek to have me
Sustain their lives

And put them
On top of the mountain
That must be conquered
Alone.

    I added the last two lines today April 16, 2006 to a poem I wrote in January of 1996. Interestingly London preceded Rachel just like some of my other writing preceded my Parkinson's disease. Layers of life removed by delving into the past.

    Tasting bits of my life at other junctures delights me now. I can remember running the narrow roads in Surrey. I remember the woods and the meadows. Ahhh. So delightful.

    However, those past moments are gone and my goal remains to write now. I wrote this recently on my blog:

The New Pastorela

Once upon a time an urban legend passed from cab driver to cab driver. "She will come just before the world is about to destroy itself and everything will change." "Watch for the light in the sky and the Shepards." "Her touch will change everything and when she comes we will pass her touch throughout the world."

Those were snippets of conversation I heard over the past few years while riding cabs. Every time I asked the cab driver about the radio transmission he would just shrug his shoulders and say, "Just some crazy cab driver talking." However, I kept hearing similar statements in other cabs. That was when I began to suspect something was happening. So I began to search. I had an FBI friend who had played baseball with me a long time ago. I asked him about urban legends. He knew I was a struggling writer looking for work, so he had pity on me and gave me some stories.

One of those stories piqued my interest and sounded similar to the snippets of conversations I heard in the cabs. It was a story about a woman who people believed would be born to lead the world to peace. I asked my friend to tell me more than his brief synopsis and he said, "Stay away from that story; I should not have started telling you about it." I asked why and he said it was because he was investigating the story. So I asked why. He told me we are always investigating these subversive stories about religious fanatics.

I stopped talking about the story and we went on drinking beer. When I flew home to Denver I never imagined that this urban legend would change my life. But it did. In the airport in a gift shop I looked at the CDs available and one of them was from a punk rock band named the Shepards. I bought the CD.

To be continued

So I have started my Pastorela story and there remains much to write on this Easter Sunday night in Denver. My right knee is killing me with pain sitting at the computer but I am driven to scribble. Why do I scribble? I search for me. I search for stories. I search for answers. Soon in this writing I hope the answers will begin to reveal themselves. This journal shall be my coming-of-age story, coming of age as a writer. This story is a birthing story with starts and stops. This story may be my story of Mara told from her slave writer's perspective. Arthur Miller married Marilyn Monroe and I shall marry Mistress Mara.

So now I shall sleep and at 6:00 am run with Brenda who is my trainer and rapidly becoming a super model.

I just noticed an e-mail from my sister that I had not read. It reminds me of the farm life in Kansas I left behind.

HI to all,

We have had a lot of snow- and wind with it- so we have some huge drifts. No school yesterday or today. With school closed, the piles of grain on the ground outside the elevator are ski mountains for the kids.

Janet.

Chapter Twenty-One
April 17, 2006

7:06 a.m. I just finished a walk/run with my trainer-confidante Brenda. We went around Cheesman Park and I had one good run but walked about half the distance. I told her about dinner with Gray and Natalia and Mara and me. I told her how I believe Mara could be an actress and a writer despite her lack of education. Brenda told me how her sister has just a high school education but is very smart and has found enormous success in New York.

One side comment before I focus. I found this scribbling from November:

November 7, 2005

> I give advice to others about their writing and stories. Start using your own advice. Write. Spend the hours you have been spending on the internet writing.

> He wrote those words and then examined them. Turned them in his hand. Blew on them to see if they would disappear like dust. He stopped typing for a moment, shook his head and said, "What is, is. The time gone is gone. Stay in the moment and write. You have dipped into the cesspool of life and the

stench of life makes your writing interesting to others.

So write. Write of what is and what has happened and what might have happened.

The jeep owner saying that jeeps are not for families; jeeps are barely sufficient to carry camping gear into the woods. He loves his straight stick dilapidated jeep though. He offers that you can mount a luggage rack on top and hook the bikes to the back.

Now to sleep.

So that was my writing before I bought a Jeep.

Last night I found Arthur Miller's autobiography, Timebends. He was married to Marilyn Monroe for a short while. A writer married to a sex idol.

I am Mistress Mara's writer but our marriage will be for life.

Chapter Twenty-Two
12:49 a.m. April 18, 2006

I know it is late and I have a brief to finish tomorrow. However, I just talked to Mara on the telephone for an hour. She called me on the downstairs telephone and I stumbled downstairs to answer it. Then I lay on the couch and talked to her about numerous topics but we got off on a discussion about prison. She spent two years in the women's penitentiary and seven months in solitary lock down with a pit to go to the bathroom in.

She said she wanted to die. She told her mother and her mother told the county officials she was suicidal and they put her in a Velcro suit.

She said she robbed banks because she was afraid to kill herself even though she was so unhappy with her life.

I will make her life into a movie. I shall be known as Mistress Mara Secret's biographer.

5:03 a.m. The pain exudes from my nipples for I am wearing her nipple clamps and I am tied to the computer table by my nipple chain. She bought me little nipple bells so she can hear me move about. I am not wearing them now but I think of Mistress's enjoyment when she gave them to me. Last night Mara dropped tacos off to me at the office when she picked up keys to our rental for her work. I spent a 475 deposit and 1200 on the first month of rent for a two bedroom apartment at Pennwood Place. Mara will work there and she is excited about it. I came up with a story about remodeling my loft which is somewhat true—I intend to put in a Jacuzzi and perhaps a new floor.

Without having Mara here I cannot wear the nipple clamps long; when she is with me and we are playing she not only has me wear them, she pulls on them and hears me moan. She tells me, "Moan like the little fuck bitch you are."

7:15a.m.   I should have run this morning because I want to weigh 180 or 175 and play with Mara. I need to get waxed as well. Then I will be a thin smooth bitch boy for her. I am amazed at her love for me in my overweight condition but then Mara does not necessarily like the young and thin and beautiful. It cannot hurt to get to thin and sexy though and still have my mind. What Mara is looking for in me is stability and to build a family? It helps that I am as sexually freaky as her. But there is more, much more to our relationship. She told me last night that she always had a high IQ but could not pay attention.

I laid back down and slept so now I must do some workout. Yet I stop to read a book that I bought years ago, "Coming of Age." His introduction made me cry several times. When art makes me cry it is good. He dedicated the book "To those old ones who still battle dragons." He quoted George Bernard Shaw: "I am of the opinion that my life belongs to the whole community and as long as I live, it is my privilege to do for it what I can. I want to be thoroughly used up when I die, for the harder I work, the more I live. I rejoice in life for its own sake. Life is no brief candle for me. It is sort of a splendid torch which I have got hold of for a moment and I want to make it burn as brightly as possible before handing it on to future generations."

I love writers. Mara will probably excel as a writer. She told me last night that she had to overcome a shyness but that she had written journals and dark poetry as a youth. Her mind organizes events and people and her things. She owns me body and soul and I am hers to organize.

Scribbling has eaten away my time. Now I must go scribble a brief. But before I stop I must dedicate myself today to writing and learning from those writers I love and others I learn to love. I want to write amusing, cutting, scripts for Mara to deliver with her blond-turned-to-dom character. Ones where men stare at her boobs only to end up staring at the floor.

Brenda, my trainer, sent me a video of Michael J. Fox talking about Parkinson's disease and acting and his efforts to help others with Parkinsons find a cure. It was inspiring and scary; his dedication was inspiring, his fidgeting scary because that is my future.

Purpose. I have purpose. Go for it now. Let this journal now reflect the Change part of the title. It was almost as if I turned giddy for a few days after turning fifty. Now, with passion and persistence I will achieve enormous change. Writing and the theater will form the basis for change. I shall succeed and Mara and I will be swept away laughing in the flood of life and fulfillment we create for ourselves. I focus and with focus I can do anything.

11:59 pm. Just before midnight. I have been working with Janice to revise the brief opposing a Motion for Summary Judgment. I have renewed my faith that I can write a brief better than anyone in this office IF, AND ONLY IF, I FOCUS. The problem has been a lack of focus and letting other matters interfere. That is why Shane bristles when he works on a brief. He understands the need for absolute focus.

Actually working with Janice has been very productive. The participation of another person keeps me focused and alert. She had me go take a nap earlier this evening and it made all the difference. Now I consider riding my bike home just to get the exercise.

Rachel called this evening to thank me for getting her through the hard times. Evidently she has some possibility of employment now. She is also refinancing her house and she says I may get some money out of that. Mara keeps spending; I sat with her in the conference room yesterday and told her that I loved her even though she spends so much money. She said, "I spend lots of money and make lots of money." Some day she will support me I am sure.

Consider words. Consider flying streamers of sentences across the page announcing the coming of a writer. This writer who shall study Arthur Miller and Camus and Tom Robbins and John Gardner and still maintain his (my) voice. My snickers shall emanate across the page, suddenly heard out loud as the typed words reach publication in the public eye.

Mistress Mara I am your writer and your husband and never shall we part and never shall I do anything to let us part. Bound by my heart and soul to hers and bound by my chains hooked to the bars of my cage I live with and for Mistress.

So the focus has come and here are my goals. Marriage, theater, out of debt entirely, yes entirely, write my way out of debt with plays, movies, books and essays. Create characters charming and crudely cavorting across the canvas of my page. Caring for all and capturing the moments.

Chapter Twenty-Three
April 20, 2006

4:41a.m. I am at the office working on the response to a Motion for Summary Judgment. Goal for the future – work out later in the day when my mind is less sharp—write early in the morning. LOL. I guess I have been writing since 2am.

Chapter Twenty-Four
April 21, 2006

    1:39 a.m. I hear Woooooooooooo outside my my third floor window—people are leaving the night club next door to my loft. I have turned on my cam as I write; it shows the lower part of my face and my sleeveless white t-shirt clad torso as I write. I have been writing a brief for three days instead of writing this journal although I wrote in my notebook last night at a restaurant.

    Yesterday I felt emotion well up against the internal walls of my body when Jenny, my secretary, told me they gave her mother two hours to live. The emotion rises again as I let my thoughts stray to Jenny and her mother who is dying. They were not ready for the reality of life. Am I? Perhaps because I have experimented with so much I am closer to ready; I remember the two dreams recently in which death was close. In one I reached the vortex of death, accepted my death and then woke.

    Trevor tells me he has spent hours studying how to cure my Parkinson's with alternative healing. We will meet this morning at a coffeeshop and I am considering giving this journal to Rita to read. I should type in the parts from my notebook.

    The blue light blinks on my tiny one gigabyte hard drive in a stick and somehow it tells me I must write. Writing while on cam is an interesting exercise in concentration. I must learn discipline in writing and eating and working out. The other thing is to clean my house and office so they are immaculate and without distractions. Then work and writing are easy. No more late night eating. In order to make my weaknesses my strengths whenever I feel like eating at night I shall work out or go for a walk. I will let myself drink liquids and that is all.

Discipline and focus. Get it now. In life and in my writing. Tailor sentences with sharp scissors, needle and thread. Create sentences that cut the consciousness and convey in structure the mood of the moment. Long languid sentences, stretched over warm days of early summer, convey a relaxed writer playing with words on a beach. Short choppy bits of thoughts, convey anxiousness and tension.

Battles come anew. Law gives me life games to play. Conditioning makes me the player others fear. Writing gives me consciousness. Writing creates something from nothing. Writing makes the ephemeral concrete. Written thoughts are eternal. That does not make them meaningful. Instead many thoughts written elicit the internet chatroom phrase that goes here: LOL….laughing out loud.

Jenny's mother dying; I relearn the practice of law; my niece graduates from college; I write briefs for filing in Chicago; an alternative healer creates a cure for my Parkinson's disease; I observe Michael J. Fox on video on the internet sent to me by my trainer who is becoming a supermodel; I am engaged to an gorgeous dominatrix who loves to fasten nipple clamps on me while wearing fashion shoes and sling cutesy purses over her shoulder; images of old times and thin body; running in the park at sunrise and a girl saying good job when I huff my thick body up the hill; midnight spoonfuls of peanut butter; typing words on a page; remembering the first time I typed words on a computer screen in a store maybe 25 years ago; thinking of the thousands of typed pages typed or dictated by me; and anticipating the coming day—the emotions—the moments—the people—Rita, Janice, Trevor, Hussein, Cheryl, Mara my love, voices—listen to them and hear the emotion and respond. Now I sleep briefly it is 3:20 a.m. Discipline in writing and body!!!!! 175 conditioned like a rock!!!! Make it happen.

6:50am.

>I made it through the night
>Sometimes that's quite a fight
>Goblins gambled golden coins
>Emboldened by the old ones
>Setting odds on my survival
>With each moments arrival
>I made it through the night
>Sometimes that's quite a fight
>With the witches sly convention
>Of spinning wicked wants of invention
>Till I scream of my perdition
>And wake once again to my condition.

Chapter Twenty-Five
Saturday April 22, 2006

2:41 a.m. Sometimes I feel as if the city embraces me. Tonight (actually Friday night) I was sitting at a table at the Blake Street Tavern with my associate attorneys Cheryl and Sam and a former client saw me, said hello and embraced me. I had represented him in the late 1980's on a large discrimination lawsuit. Sometimes the past meets the present.

5:35 a. m. I am going downstairs to take a dose of the flower potion given to me by Trevor yesterday morning to cure the Parkinson's. Also I will buy blueberries and eat a half cup of them per day. Blueberries and flower potions – why not take a chance to get healed.

I save this writing and the blue light of my tiny hard drive flashes at me. Yesterday was a momentous day, a delightful day and a sad day. The sadness came when I found out late in the day that Jenny's Mother died at 7 a.m. Janice called me on my cell and told me that Jenny had emailed the news. I will take flowers to her home today.

May Sarton wrote journals. I wonder where I put her journal that I was reading?

1:45 P.M. Rachel keeps trying to get me to come over to her house. I just read her email to me yesterday.

I just spoke with you this Friday morning. Although I was more so doing my 'laugh yelling', I still deem your behavior as UNACCEPTABLE. I think I am pretty accepting and understanding of a lot of things that have been thrown my way, but the idea of YOU not coming over to spend good time, at this lovely house is UNACCEPTABLE.

Honestly, I understand the control thing and all that, but I also know there are boundries and safe words. So please tell Miss Thang, that the boundry is true and real friendship and the safe word is 'bite me' – says me!

This is a great movie here (Tully) and I (despite popular belief) am a true and good friend and I'll be here long after whats-her-name has come and gone...

Second Appeal: (All honesty and normality aside) ....LIE! Yep. Just lie. and be good at it. AND (here's the good part) confess and be punished! It's a 'win-win' situation. Tell her you're going to a theatre meeting. Come over, watch the movie, have a nice time, then tell her you've been a bad boy... could be a lot of fun.

Third Appeal: (The basic facts) Tell her that her thinking, on this is wrong. As long as you are happy and she is above board, it's fantastic! I am happy for the both of you (truly) and there is no need for silliness. She can come along for the movie and cook out too.

Bottom Line: I'm going to be here for a long time, whether she is or not, and I think this childish turf thing is silly, at best. She will too, when she realizes that I'm no threat and all for it, if it's making you happy.

one last note.

I have wood tools here.
big saws, drills and things.

> I have resisted going over to Rachel's house.

Chapter Twenty-Six
April 23, 2006

1:30 a.m. I am tremendously happy. Mara and I spent the night together. We shopped at the Overland store in LoDo and I did not buy the Chinchilla coat that was 5700 dollars although I was tempted to do so. I did spend 600 plus dollars there and 900 at Fascinations and I gave Mara 700 in cash. We are going to get married there is no question in my mind. I showed Mara the email of Rachel and she was happy with me for doing that and her comment was that Rachel was the one being childish and she had her chance. We ended the night at the apartment at Penwood Place where Mistress tightened my nipple clamps and beat my ass with the riding crop and did something new. She choked me with a rope. I begged to see her breasts and she showed them to me and smothered me with them and choked me and then I came incredibly.

I want to swim there in the morning. I need to get my goggles from the office.

Now to bed and sleep well.

7:00 a.m. I have been puttering around the house printing pictures of Mara, trying to put them in frames, thinking about things and now I'm using Dragon speak to start writing again. All of a sudden I have charged up my credit card so that I only have a few thousand dollars of credit left and only a few dozen dollars left in the bank. I did put $5,000 in the Blues House account which makes a difference. I spent $450 a month no actually $560 a month in storage costs. I've hired Becky full-time to do the running with respect to the theater because I can't and still make a living. I have helped out Jack with cash of $400 and I helped out Greg not only with four hundred dollars for a monthly payment but also with a few hundred dollars to fix his truck. I helped out Rachel when she asked for $1500. Mara has taken thousands of dollars; I don't keep track of that precisely because she will be my wife, but she's very expensive. She says we will be all right and I hope so. In any case, what is mine is hers and that's the way it is.

Last night we spent $60 on the carriage ride, $660 at the Overland store in Lower downtown and we spent almost $1000 at Fascinations an adult store. I gave her $700 dollars. Mara got a leather hood for me; she got a bridle for me; she got a little couch with restraints which she's going to use to restrain me so I cannot move and in the fuck me like the slut I am. My cock gets hard thinking about the fact that I am owned by a dominatrix who loves to fuck me with a strap on. Interesting I suddenly remember a hotel room in which a young escort came back for the second time after she bought a strap on; it had a vibrator. She fucked me very hard and I think I bled afterwards. Now, I am Mara's slut. She got a big cock and a new harness last night and told me that today she will fuck me. She tells me she loves it when I whimper and she makes me whimper with pain. Last night I was totally in her control. She down bound by wrists together and put two sets of nipple clamps on my nipples and used a riding crop on my ass and a rope around my neck.

Now in the moment thinking about last night I fasten nipple clamps to my nipples that have weights on them. My cock is so hard I want to be at her feet sucking her toes to feeling her pull on the nipple clamps so hard so that I scream in pain. I love Mistress and she owns me.

8:20 a.m. I think I only slept a few hours and I am running out of time to work out and to write and to take flowers to Jenny and to meet with Jack, Greg and Dana and Becky. Greg does not want Damin Daren on the board of directors for the nonprofit, but I do. And I want people who are in my court because I do not want to be liable for all the costs of the theater and have no control.

I have to get myself to 180 stay there and get married.

Chapter Twenty-Seven
Monday, April 24, 2006

8:00 a.m. Focus and get to the office and then write. Go!!!!

9:10 a.m. I must focus myself. Yesterday I took flowers to Jenny and her husband and had a long talk with them in their living room. They had been sitting on the floor sorting papers of her mom. I suggested she call a probate attorney and get some advice as to what to do as executor of her mother's estate.

5:50 PM. This is a test of the rainfall forest monitoring system for primitive rain forests in Brazil.

Chapter Twenty-Eight
Tuesday April 25, 2006

1:43 a.m. I found this quote of my writing on a blog on an alternative life style site. I am toxic.

Quoting toxic:

Discovery in yourself is wonderful, however discovery in a person you have taught is exhilarating because it means they have opened your gift and used it.

toxic

Magnificent comment! So accurate, and you present this statement like a red carpet rolling out.

Perfection in language, I do so enjoy words! lol

Hugs,
Savanna

Written for Mistress just now and posted on the blog.

Find words and juggle them till they please the eye, but keep the eye on the kaleidoscope least it dissolve into falling balls.

Mistress you are my muse and my chaos. My muse masters me and makes me want to write miraculous stories that both amuse and bring the meltdown into tears. And from chaos comes extreme creativity.

All I write derives from your love for me and my love for you and our friendship in both caress and pain.

You make me yours and I make you mine and together we blend our mind and soul. Your command comes from my desires and my desires arise from your imagination till one merges into the other and we are a multicolored ball rolling down the hill of life so fast we scarce can breath with the excitement of love rolled into one.

I rewrote the prelude to my blog as well. Now it reads:

The mist that changes all has obscured my floor. Words, thoughts made real, part the mist so I, and you with me, may view the depths beneath my floor, under which, you find my soul.

I also commented on Mistress Savanna's angry outburst on her blog and she quoted me,

Quoting toxic:

As an outsider--I have rare visitors to my humble blog--I have no clue about who runs what on blogville but I do know that I love your love of words and language Mistress and when you are angry I love the steam that rises from your blog to the world (above?)... better said the steam that engulfs the world...Mistress I hope this day betters the last and words of anger turn to amusing ridicule of subs who have lost the understanding that without full submission they cannot experience the love that only comes from complete immersion. Now they are but chattering humans wishing for that which they have lost by their own noise.

She quoted me and then said, "Dear toxic,

I think that you are not an outsider, but a true insider. *wink*. I think that I shall also have to pay some regular visits to your blog, because you make Me smile with these words.

Absolutely spectacular comprehension of servitude, spoken with these words: "Mistress I hope this day betters the last and words of anger turn to amusing ridicule of subs who have lost the understanding that without full submission they cannot experience the love that only comes from complete immersion. Now they are but chattering humans wishing for that which they have lost by their own noise."

I think, I may decide to simply stick to male submissives from this point. Lol."

Hugs and kisses,

Mistress Savanna

Then she visited my blog and said,

Dear toxic,

your Mistress is very lucky indeed. If She has trained you, I applaud Her. I wish you both the best in this world and I hope that your love for each other continues to grow and flourish.

My regards to your Mistress M., She has My respect.

Hugs,

Mistress Savanna

Fifty and change. Mara is the first love of my life—the only love of my life.

8:00 a.m.

What will this day bring. I have only done floor exercises; I cannot walk to work because I am scheduled to meet Marvin for coffee at 11:00a.m. I must move quickly now, but consider the night—my writing was complemented by a blog writer that I follow a bit, Mistress Savanna.

Time passes; it is still the first month and the 25th day of my first year—saying I am one again. Perhaps I shall call this my second childhood, perhaps everyone should count themselves lucky at reaching fifty and start their adult childhood at age fifty.

Mara will turn twenty-five in September and be half my age. She struggles for adulthood sometimes, but mostly that comes from the perception created by her mother to hold her down. The most interesting aspect of yesterday was the unsolicited comment by Alice that we should get together and play scrabble this week. I look forward to seeing and hearing her poetry and rap and hip hop. Her garb of young black boy gangster and her sunglasses and steady cool masks her character and makes me so curious to find the writer inside. The 24-year-old writer who probably has fucked Mara with a strap on. Just a guess. Certainly they have made love.

Find the stories today!!!! Go.

Sam asked for vacation and I replied:

Vacation?

Problems arise unexpectedly in the middle of the night
So the very moment you are out of sight
The partners will flip on their shrouded light

And look about for an associate to join the fight

Noticing only then you are gone they prate it just aint right.

So slip away quietly and smugly take your flight

To parts unknown

And might I suggest,

Leave your phone

Sitting at home.

Chapter Twenty-Nine
April 26, 2006

1:09 a.m. Once again money makes me think that I am just a fool, that I am being played for a fool. Today Mara had me get her 2000 dollars after I gave her 700 on Saturday and 300 yesterday. She maxed out the other credit card again after I have paid it down twice at least. I explained the dire financial straits and she had me get 2000 dollars for her in part to pay for the advertisement. Should I try to buy the duplex for her business or should I simply stop spending? I am tired. I shall sleep and consider all this again later.

I am going to do a 4pm diet. After 4 pm I shall only eat fruits and vegetables and drink juices. Run at 5 am tomorrow. 180 as soon as possible. Focus focus focus.

I must lose 60 lbs. as soon as possible. Now I am dictating to Sajina and suddenly the words appear on the screen quickly and accurately. I'm no longer hampered by misconstruction of words. I can dictate sentence is very quickly and accurately if I say the words right.

A patent attorney I know called me about a case yesterday which is very important to him. They have been looking for investors all over the country. It was a case that he won $20 million and then lost on appeal. It requires an incredible investment of time and money but there is a potential recovery of millions. It is time to start playing the game, to get the body in shape and the voice in shape because shortly I'm going to be going to trial in many trials and I must get my sharpness back. I must work out every day hard and kept in to work early.

I must be wrong about Mara. She loves me. I wish it with all my heart. I hope I am more than just a source of money.

I hate it when she finds a new girl and never calls me. It makes me think that I am a man and she loves women. Anyway I'm tired and I'm thinking crazy and I need to go to bed and go to sleep and wake up fine forgetting all of these strange thoughts.

Yesterday my writing was lyrical and complimented by Mistress Savanna who is an intense writer of blogs on. Why do I need compliments? They certainly give you the quiet warmth of satisfaction.

I must write about Greg Berge. But I'm too tired right now and it is almost 2 am. If I intend to me my goals for tomorrow I need to sleep and sleep well.

Ultimately, the theater is my work of art. But more important than the theater is my relationship with Mara. I love her purely and dearly but she spends so fucking much money. Oh well. Money is money. Love is something entirely different and I love Mara. End of chapter. It is time to close the book on this tired refrain.

1:51 am. I'm still writing and I'm going to transcribe a few paragraphs from the notebook to the page so that it is all in one place. The "it" if refer to is Fifty and Change this book that is being written by me almost involuntarily.

Chapter Thirty
April 27, 2006

12:26 p.m. We have worked on creating a theater. Now I am flat broke it seems and the dream is both close and distant.

5:03 p.m. So my money situation is critical. Mara has taken thousands of dollars for her daughter's daycare, for advertisements, for buying outfioo my fingers cannot stop from holding down a key because my brain is just shutting off over and again. I have 3300 dollars in the bank and I have to pay $1500 down on thoooooooooooooooooooooooooooooooooooooooooooooooooooooooooooooooooooooooooooooooooooooooooooooooooooooooooooooooooooooooooooooooooooooooooooooooooooooooooooooooooooooooooooooooooooooooooooooo on the duplex that will be turned into a dungeon. Mara is not earning money and I have none. So much for the 50000 she was going to create out of the 10,,,lllllllllllllllllllllllllllllllllllllllllllllllllllllllllllllllllllllllllllllllllllllllllllll ten thousand that I gave her. But instead I have spent another ten thousand on her. I am so tired. I need to finish the complaint for Nadine. This typing looks just like my mind feels.

Chapter Thirty-One
April 28, 2006

7:10 am. It was raining outside at 5:30 a.m. when I started to walk for morning walk/run around Cheesman. On Wednesday I had left my heart monitor at the apartment at Pennsylvania Place. No. 1400 that we rented so that Mara would have a place to work. I decided to detour slightly and pick up my heart monitor and watch. Mara had been working last night but my guess was that she was gone so I went upstairs in the elevator and put my key in the lock. It had passed through my mind as to how upset I would be if Mara were in the apartment sleeping with some guy. I turned the key and pushed the door in and it was barricaded. I pushed harder and then pulled it shut and locked it. I knocked when I heard someone on the other side. Eventually after I said, "It is Stephan," Mara opened the door. I said that I came to get my heart monitor. She turned and went to get it and when she came back I said, "Can I come in?" She said no and I said who is there and she said Alice but she is asleep. I was angry but I said nothing except, "Ok." I turned on my heel and left. Many thoughts ran through my mind on my walk back to the loft. I considered going running……

I have to go meet with Trevor.

10:56 a.m. When I got to the office, Jimmy Dice left a message that he had to cancel on lunch and so I will not be able to find out if he is still ok with lending $50,000 dollars to me. I wrote a check for the escrow on Becky's duplex (one side of it) and that reduced the account below the amount needed to cover my house payment which is automatically drawn on the 5th of the month. However, Janice said that she would cut me a check for $5000 dollars today even though she wouldn't be able to fully calculate the numbers for distribution. So I will put that in my account for now. At least I thought she would do that; now she tells me my account is negative.

I digress for a moment. Last night I signed the purchase documents for the duplex, the place that will make a perfect dungeon for Mara. Then I went to a refuge place run by a nonprofit where a woman I know teaches poetry to at-risk youth. Another friend of my friend was there. It was a low turnout night and the kids who were left, left early to go see Othello at the Denver Center. In the end it was three of us. We chatted but before we went my friend had us write and I wrote a poem that was to be a person speaking form a position of power but not control. I wrote the following in the three-minute limit:

The lights went out

And the sounds of bubbles

Stayed in my ears.

The luminescence sparkles

When cut by fins that shear

Through water currents

cold and warm and cold again.

We surface,

 holding each other to find,

Our faces beneath the moon

And we turn to each other

And say, "I love you."

This morning I considered running after encountering the barricaded door, but realized that I wanted to talk to Mara and I did not have my telephone. I walked back to the loft considering the meaning of the barricaded door. Was there another guy in there? Was there drugs strewn across the table? Was she sleeping with Alice? Should I end our relationship? Should I be mad or sad or accept that she did not trust me enough to tell me the truth? When I arrived at the Loft, the Loft that yesterday I determined to sell because selling it would enhance my relationship with Mara, basically throwing me into the mix of life—I would live at the Pennsylvania Street apartment—I still did not know what I would say to Mara.

Honesty. That is all I want and the barricaded door told me that Mara does not trust me and was hiding something. Or at least that is how it seems. Since she has never stayed a single entire night with me I wonder. Does she just make love to women these days.

Does she do crack or meth or ecstasy? Actually one time she had remarked that she had been on ecstasy when she visited me at the office. So when I reached the loft I saw that Mara had called three or four times and sent three or four text messages to me in the time it took to walk a few blocks. The text messages had come after the missed calls.

Chapter Thirty-Two
Saturday April 29, 2006

10:30 a.m. Yesterday morning at 5:40 a.m.I walked back in the rain to find my phone filled with text messages and missed calls. It is hard to believe it was only yesterday morning. And I only had to walk a few blocks back from Pennsylvania. Let me see--- there was Grant street, Logan Street, Sherman Street, Lincoln and Broadway. Then I was home to the loft that I said I was going to sell to be with Mara. Now I was uncertain about everything.

I looked at the phone messages which came after the three missed phone calls. The first three said, "I really don't feel like going through this again--answer your phone or call me, Alice is my friend and I'm not going to startle her, just like I wouldn't let someone come in the house while u are sleeping I had a session late last night and didn't wanna drive home if you could only trust me if you're gonna flip out lemme kno and all have my sister come get her table and all take my stuff this is fucked."

The next message said,

"Lemme kno when you wanna take my truck back. Lmao…. You r confused."

I dialed Mara's phone number and it played the Donald Trump ego thing to the end and then the messages were full. I dialed again and no answer again. Finally, on the third time she answered and I told her that I loved her and that I was not freaking out and that she shouldn't go off on me. She was surprised, totally surprised.

When I got home, even before I saw the messages, I knew this was a huge turning point in our relationship. It was either over or it would be stronger. I hoped that she had called, because if she had not called then I would not know what to do. But Mara had called repeatedly and I knew she cared and I knew I was hopelessly in love with her even if she had been sleeping with Alice or another guy or whatever. Hopelessly is not the right word. I am in love with Mara and it is unlike any love I have ever known. My ass is black and blue from her beating me with her strap. I sucked her toes Wednesday night as she talked on the telephone and then she had me use the suction cup dildo on the wall and fuck myself for her viewing pleasure.

When she left the message she did not even consider that the truck was at a repair shop and I was the only one who could get it out. Yesterday I could have picked up the truck from the repair place myself if I had freaked out but I did not even consider it. I want to marry Mara and live with her and make our lives grow together.

However, I decided against selling the loft. If I cannot go into an apartment I am renting I am not going to sell my home. I guess I will hedge just a bit. If anything it can be used for rehearsal space and an office for the theater.

9:20 p.m. Mara called me today upset because her phone wasn't charging and had me spend more money, this time on a Blackberry phone for her. This because it would take four to six weeks to get her a new sidekick phone. I am already paying for one extra phone that Alice uses. The Blackberry is suppose to be the family only number and keep the minutes down but we will see.

So I sat down to write after seeing Tully. Mara had told me to get Rachel's phone back so I went over and saw the movie that Rachel had wanted me to watch. Her male friend showed up in the middle and so it was hard to experience the movie which was excellent. I had to fight back tears on several occasions. I believe it was filmed in Nebraska and it was a farm story. There was some transparency in the plot but on the whole the movie was moving.

Yesterday, Friday the 28th of April was momentous for completely unexpected reasons. I expected to have lunch with Jimmy Dice who had offered to lend me 50,000 dollars which is sorely needed but he called and canceled. I expected to have a decision in on the appeal but it did not get issuedsddddddddddddddddddddddddddddddddddddddddddddddddddd dddddddddddddddddddddddddddddddddddddddddddddddddddddddd dddddddddddddddddddddddddddddddddddddddddddddddddddddddd ddddddddddddddddddd damn the Parkinson's took over my brain and finger control again and I held down the "d" for a moment or two.

What about my relationship with Mara? She has spent close to $150,000 of my money in less than a year; otherwise I could finance the theater without a doubt. And I still love her; she is my mistress and my friend although the barricade at the Pennsylvania Street door and her constant need to spend money on something even when I tell her I am flat broke. A few days ago she was promoting buy inaaaaaaaaaaaaaaaaaaaaaaaaaaaaaaaaaaaaaaaaaaaaaaaaaaaaaaaa aaaaaaaaaaaaaaaaaaaaaaaaaaaaaaaaaaaaaaaaaaaaaaaaaaaaaaaaaa aaaaaaaaaaaaaaaaaaaaaaaaaaaaaaaaaaaaaaaaaaaaaaaaaaaaaaaaaa aaaaaaaaaaaaaaaaaaaaaaaaaaaaaaaaaaaaaaaaaaaaaaa D am I hate Parkinsons and the feeling of lost moments. See ablvell

Ok, start again. It is 9:45 and I don't want to forget the events of yesterday, but I need a short nap.

11:14 p.m. I just got off the phone with Mara who called me to say hello. The landlord came by and said the sprinkler system doesn't work. He supposedly is going to get some estimates. Mara says she likes the house and wants to live there for a while.

The backyard is a mess, as is the front yard. However, I have not seen the house since I saw it when it was initially leased. Mara has not allow me to come over. I hope that someday she feels comfortable with me and truly lets me into her life. I admit that I have been somewhat flaky in the past, but that was the past. She should view Friday morning as the ultimate test of me. I accepted what she said and did not blow up or lose my cool. I left when she would not let me in the apartment, but I did not blow my cool. If she is lying to me so be it, I accept it and hope that she will change. I will believe her no matter what because she is my mistress and I accept her word. Soon she will realize that I am her friend, lover, husband, partner for life. I am risking all I have in life because I love her.

Now I remember when I spoke to her yesterday morning after I returned to the loft, I was crying because I love her so much. And now I will be confident in my love. I will not need to question her or question whether she trusts me. When I go to the apartment I will knock as instructed. I do not plan on being there often, but I do want to swim in the morning.

I just put Quidam music in the DVD player. Quidam was the Cirque du Soleil show that was both ambiguous and delightful.

Yesterday was momentous for another reason. I went to celebrating a new musical. I was only going to stay for an hour and then go. Instead I was charmed by Jason again and then played two hours of tennis, including an entire set. In the process I met, a fiftyish woman tennis pro and learned more intriguing facts about Jason. He is very competitive.

I also met an old Italian executive, who is friends with friends of mine. He took the time to write down my name. He knew one of them came from a small Kansas town. He said one of my friends was turning 65 and knew someone very active in the theater scene.

Who else did I meet? A musically inclined accountant, a musically inclined camera person, and an oversized ex-Buddist monk.

And then there was Mistress Mara. She grows her wings with me. I am her slave and will be her strongest supporter forever. Mara is her given name and she has served prison time for two or three – I think three felonies. She has told me stories of prison that I need to get in more detail, including reading the Bible three times and smuggling pot into prison in her pussy.

What I expected to happen yesterday did not happen: I did not get comments on the theater lease and I did not get the valuation of the land in Kansas which will hopefully give me financial security for the near future. I borrowed 150,000 on it last year and used much of it to pay off my accumulated credit card debt. It could be worth 490000 dollars based on the land market.

Playwriting idea: take online profiles and write a play with those characters. I met with Trevor and Becky today and saw the inside of Cervantes. There was a jazz festival going at Five Points. I cannot wait to have the theater running. It will do well.

Chapter Thirty-Three
April 30, 2006

    The last day of the first month after turning fifty. I feel so alone in this loft. I know now why I wanted to sell it. Loneliness. I want to be with Mara all the time. Patience is needed. I hope I am not being deceived or this will be a sad love story. I tried to go to bed but I could only think about Mara and my loneliness. Perhaps I will work out. Mara took the call from her sister and said she was going to call back but she did not. She tells me all the time that she loves me. I love her and this journal is a strange love story playing itself out. She told me she would never throw me out.

    When we go out she often has me get on my knees in front of her and she puts nipple clamps on my nipples and tightens them down so I gasp. When we are alone and I am wearing nothing but my collar and nipple clamps Mistress will ask me who owns me and I will say, "You own me Mistress Mara." If I say it softly she will hit me with her strap or crop and ask me again and again until I scream her name and then she pulls on the nipple clamps and in my pain I tell her how much I love her. Now I sit and write naked except for a collar and cockstrap. I am hers. Now I will fasten the nipple clamps to my swollen nipples. My purpose in life is so clear when I wear her clamps. I live solely for her pleasure. Oh my god Mistress how I love you.

    12:41 I just got off the phone with Mistress. Then a fellow called about the lighting design and we discussed the theater and how much he would charge—2000-3000 dollars. First he asked what I thought was fair. I said I have never done this and then he said what he would normally would charge which was 2000 dollars and I said that was fair or 3000 was fair or whatever he thought after it was done. In the past, when he did the lighting for plays he charged a bottle of whiskey.

While I was talking to the lighting designer, I saw Rachel called. Then Brenda called and rearranged the meeting for tomorrow and I gave up my workout time at 6 am so that we can have coffee at 7 a.m. and take care of Brenda and her friend's class requirements. I called Rachel back. Oops. In between City Card called and said I was over the credit limit. However I had already set in motion an electronic payment and the person at City Card noted the fact down and told me to ignore future computer calls.

So I was going to write about was that Mistress wanted me to sign over the vehicle to her. That is, give her my Jeep Cherokee. I said I would do that but I was worried that her creditors might take it. She obviously doesn't trust me completely yet. Quite frankly, my creditors may be the ones coming after the Jeep Cherokee. I still know what ex-partner's bankruptcy trustee is going to do about his claim against his so-called partnership interest. Anyway I'm getting off the topic in the topic is that I told mistress and I would do whatever she said and I would trust her not to destroy me. So what she told me to do was transfer the truck to her and gets us a membership at the Denver athletic club. I said I would do that and I will because now I know that I am owned by her and if I cease to be her slave I will I will die if not physically then mentally. I would give up my current life and leave. I cannot imagine being without Mara. I am crying just writing these words. I need her and want her and love her and whatever she asks I will try to perform. She owns my soul. I will advise her what I think that she will make choices for us and and that is how I am going to live the rest of my life.

So now I'm going for the run. The first thing I want to do though is look at her picture and memorize each one of her tattoos and each curve of her body and the precise brown of her eyes. I'm going to remember for a few moments the feeling of her strap on cock thrusting into my man pussy and the feel of her black leather strap hitting my ass painfully as she thrusts into me. I cannot masturbate without her permission. My cock hardens thinking these thoughts. I drop my running clothes to the floor. I get her picture and sit it on the table where I'm dictating to the computer and I reach for the nipple clamps. As I hold them the chain rubs against my cock and then I open each of the clamps and place them over my nipples. I think of Mara my mistress and I release the clamps to shooting pain, excrutiating pain, incredible pain, pain that makes my cock so fucking hard. I can see myself on the bed with my ass in the air and my fiancée fucking me. Mistress Mara owns me body and soul. My life is meaningless without her. I am her slave her fuck slut who eats my own come and licks her toes when she sits on the couch and offers her feet to me. I approach her on my knees in front of the couch and as I think those thoughts of what I have done in the past, come seeps to the surface and I take my finger and wipe the come from the head of my cock and then suck my fingers. The nipple clamps dig into my nipples and I think of bringing her title to my truck in my teeth and laying it at her feet. She owns me and I am only beginning to understand the meaning of this ownership.

Now I will go for my run at 2:22 p.m. on this beautiful Sunday afternoon.

4:12 p.m. I finally got away for a run at 3 p.m. Actually it was more of a walk than a run because my legs are still incredibly stiff from the tennis match on Friday night.

The end of the month is here. My billing has been bad for the second straight month. I need to get the bills done.

The water tastes exceptionally good and I have sweat on my brow from the exercise.

Now I have more things to do from Mistress. First write some reviews for her. Then get some stuff for the apartment and throw the trash out. I need a haircut but it may not be today.

Chapter Thirty-Four
May 1, 2006

1:30 a.m. Mistress is financially destroying me, but I still love her. Yesterday afternoon she called me and had me meet her at Best Buy in Aurora. She had me use my credit card and buy her a car stereo system for 880 dollars and a new fancy dryer for 1200 dollars. That on top of a new Blackberry phone on Saturday. She said she would pay me back for the dryer and the car stereo equipment next week but Mara has never paid me back anything she has said she would over the past two years. She said that the delivery of the dryer on Tuesday would be fine even though she was working because her Mom or her sister would be at the house.

That comment triggered thoughts about her mother. I wonder at her Mother not willing to talk to me due to my relationship with Mara, but more than willing to accept the benefits of my relationship with Mara including checks directly payable to her. I think her mom demonstrates the meaning of the word "hypocrisy."

I have gone from having 30,000 in the bank and no credit card debt at the beginning of January to having maybe 2000 in the bank and 25,000 of credit card debt. Add on top of that the fact I earned 56,000, actually 61,000 since the start of the year. I gave Mara 10,000 one time, 3000 another time, 6,000 or so when she was in Vegas not counting paying her 1700 house payment each month. She probably has cost me 12000-14000 or more a month for four months. Last year I paid 26,000 for her body work alone. Unless something happens differently soon, I will be in financial ruin and have to sell the Loft and the land in Kansas and the theater will fail.

However, last night at Best Buy she made me laugh. Buying the car stereo equipment for the truck she said we are working out compromises between us: we are buying the stereo equipment for the truck instead of getting a BMW and we are joining the Denver Athletic Club at her behest and she is quitting smoking.

I love Mara and I will accept financial ruin if it comes to that, but as an alternative I am trying to make more money and raise the money for the theater which of course also contributed a great deal to the profligate spending since January.

As I consider my relationship with Mara I start to see the similarities between our physical sexual relationship and our mental and financial relationship. The conflicts between pain and ecstasy and how pain succumbs to ecstasy and although she beats me till my ass is black and blue I tell her in my pain that I love her and I do. When I met her at the store she was wearing a blue sweat suit and was stunningly beautiful. Just being with her amazes me sometimes. At the store she made me go out to my Jeep and get my collar and when I came back in wearing a leather collar with a ring on the front I spent money freely for her. Occasionally she would entwine her finger in the collar ring and pull me close and whisper that she wanted her leash. Sometimes, it seems I am living a dream. Even as I write this I realize that money means nothing when held in the light of my love for Mara. I will give freely.

After we got out of the store, Mara sat in the Jeep with me. I had her read the passage I wrote just before I went running and she liked it a lot. Then she had me put on nipple clamps. She told me that she loved me and that I made her whole while she twisted the nipple clamps. She said, "Do these make your cock hard? You know how I like that." She told me that next weekend she would find a girl for me to fuck while she watched and while I was wearing my collar and nipple clamps. She said, "You had better please her too or I will beat your ass hard." She went on, "Rub your cock for me." I rubbed my now hard cock through my thin sweats and she smiled as she watched. She twisted my clamped nipple and I gasped and began to moan as she used her iron-grip to inflict excruciating pain.

As she twisted the clamps, in her expressive little girl voice she said, "I could have you masturbate and come here in the parking lot like I did before but I want you to go home and make a video of you masturbating for me so I can watch it when I don't have the real thing." "And I want you to come and lick it up for me. Remember I am giving you permission to masturbate only if you make the video."

At the risk of understatement, my life is changing. In the middle of all of it is Mara—the chaos and the passion that is Mara—is leading me to incredible new levels of creativity. Mara makes life worth living.

A message I received from the person at whose house I played tennis yesterday and the person who created a musical:

Morning Stephan:

"Five Simple Steps to Emotional Healing". Gloria Arenson.
You are healed! As rare as it seems we get together each time we do seems to reinforce the fact that we should work together more. I want to do whatever I can to become a part of your theatre creation. Even tho you and Paula beat Alice and I!

The author I mentioned was coming to the party, had an emergency and "wired" his regrets. You will meet him soon.

I remember quite vividly, on the occasion of an earlier meeting, when after the big production number, how you were so emotional and engaged in the idea of "calming" the flow of the show at that point. Don't think I didn't notice. I also corrected that area in the new re-write.

You mentioned a play you wrote?
Count me in.

Best,
Jason

4:00 a.m. I realize that one of the next plays I need to write is a two person play between a Mistress and her submissive with separate monologues by each of them.

Chapter Thirty-Five
May 2, 2006

9:40 a.m. office. Parkinson's Disease has changed my life. It has changed the priorities in my life, the course of my life and the ease of my life. It has changed my creative output first by a long depression that I can see now only because it is gone and by the lack of mobility that makes typing or scribbling difficult.

Yesterday, the most intense moment of the day was when, while standing at the doorway to her office, I asked Jenny, my secretary, why she pulled the shades to the interior window to her office. She told me, "I break down and cry often and I don't want people to see me crying. Her mother died a week ago Friday. As she said those words she began to cry. We hugged each other for a long time.

I am dictating my bills for last month this morning and I remember how last month Jenny called me worried about me because gibberish showed up on the tape during entries. Parkinson's strikes again. Last night I slept well, but there is pressure from many sources right now and I begin to feel desperate.

Now I am to go have coffee with Marvin, who had an accident last week on the way to have coffee with me.

9:30 pm. I am here at the office because it is time that I finish some projects: I have to finish the complaint and deliver it to the client tomorrow. I'm using Dragon Speak because my hands are not typing well tonight. I am becoming more adept with Dragon Speak. That is good because there will come a time that I cannot type.

When I started this day I vowed to remember the events. Mara had asked me to take down the trash from the Pennsylvania apartment and I walked over at about 7:30 a.m. to do so. Last night I slept the best I have slept in ages. It was as though I slept three separate nights because I woke three times during the night.

I have to turn Dragon Speak off because I am not getting the words right. Typing slowly is sometimes better than speaking fast and correcting each phrase for thirty seconds.

Looking at this day backwards, running the video in reverse, I see myself sitting by the river in the dark of the evening at about 8:00 p.m. talking to Trevor on my cell phone. He is telling me about coming up with the name for the poets, actually names, "The Word Artists" and the "Denver Poetry Company."

10:39 I just spoke to Wayne, the leader of Rocky Horror Picture Show for a half hour when I did not have a half hour. He has been laid off and is looking for work. He told me his background and he has multiple history degrees. And I want historic plays to run every afternoon in the theater. Passion for history and a theatrical and teaching background makes Wayne perfect for creating another aspect of the theater that I envision... He even suggested walking tours that I quickly equated with employment for actors.

Shane Heitman actually knocked on my door and asked what was going on. He told me that a joint client wants him to replace their New York attorneys and get licensed in New York. I said that is good news and, "You shouldn't be wanting for work, then." My thought was that you will never share any of that work with me even if I am going broke but perhaps I misjudge Shane.

I need to finish the Complaint for the new client tonight. It is essential. That or in the early morning perhaps I take home the files...no it does no good I must do it here at the office but it is 11:10 p.m. Early morning is best. Tomorrow I will ride my bike in to work after I ride it home tonight.

Mara has not called tonight despite the fact she said she would call me back at 6:00 P.M. . I am not secure in knowing she loves me because I begin to believe that she has everything she wants from me and does not care. Today she called me while I was sitting at a coffeshop downtown and had me deliver my set of keys to the Pennsylvania apartment to the front desk so she could pick them up and meet a client. Now I have no keys to the apartment I have rented and I wonder if she will return them or whether she intends to not allow me to have keys to the apartment.

Now I will sit back and see what happens. I love her; I wish I were sure that she loves me for me not just for the thousands of dollars she has me spend on her. She rarely kisses me on the lips and has never slept with me in bed and I don't think any of her family knows we are engaged to be married. Will all this end when the money runs out?

The land appraised much lower that I hoped: 255,000 dollars and I have 150,000 borrowed against it. I was hoping it would appraise for 480,000 but I was wrong. Hopefully the bank will loan some more money and I can pay off my current credit card debt and buy the half duplex.

It is now 11:30 and I am tempted to turn off my cell because I begin to get the feeling that Mara only calls when she wants something from me. Will we ever see a movie together? She picked out movies for me at Target last night and then kept them. She talked to me at 9:15 pm last night and I was laying on the bed undressed and she made me dress and come to Target and buy 900 dollars worth of stuff even though she knew I was broke and had little credit left.

I am tired. Go home and sleep. Don't be insecure. If she doesn't love you, she doesn't. If she loves you it is wonderful. I tanned today at about 5:45. There were an incredible number of girls who showed up to tan. If you are ever looking again remember the gaggle of girls with great variety.

Also remember the beauty of sitting by the river with the lights playing off the ripples and currents. And remember the contrasts of talking to a financial broker and a theater person together at coffee. I invited Jake to our play reading on May 10. The financial broker wore a suit and a tie and told about his accident a week ago on his way to have coffee with me. I think the theater person will make a difference. I am collecting a real team to make this theater happen.

The question I must answer is whether I am going to Washington D.C. for my niece's graduation.

Fund raising!!!!!!

Chapter Thirty-Six
May 3, 2006

This is going to be one fucking difficult day. I did not sleep last night, at least not more than an hour. I kept debating whether to come into the office or to try sleep a few more hours. I succeeded in neither although I am the first person in the office at a little before 8 AM. I rode my bike into work; at least I have worked out for the day. When I arrived at the office door there was a very large older white woman looking for a key which she didn't have. I got off my bicycle and untangled the briefcase strap that I was fighting the entire ride and dug out my keys. I said, "A man with the keys." She laughed, and I went on and said, "There are so few that have keys today." She said, "What did you say?" I said, "Oh, I was just being poetic." She said, "Oh." When we got to the elevator as I was holding my bicycle, I said, to myself, but also to her, "There are keys to rainy days like today, there are keys to sunny days like yesterday and there are keys to the river below, but so few have keys anymore." She said, "Yes, that is true, I am going to have to ask Jenny for a key." I sighed. She got off on floor two and I kept going up. There was a guy on the elevator who was onboard when the woman and I entered. The elevator was acting quite slow and the guy was drinking coffee. I said, as we finally arrived at the third floor, "The elevator acts as if it needs coffee too." He laughed. At least he got the joke. Perhaps early morning poetry is like drinking; people just don't think it's right.

1:43 p.m. A poet friend of mine responded to the above "poem" when I sent it to him by sending the following:

> what's right is right
> what's nothing is something
> what's what but a word
>
> what's that space between the lines

what's that space between my thoughts

yogurt granola coffee

it'll be a good afternoon! - ever heard the cure song strange day?

    I sent an email to the poet that Cheryl was going to download the song for me. I've been working with Cheryl to revise a litigation brief. I came up with some points she had not thought about.

    This morning Cheryl and I met with two persons from my business plan class, about trademarks and copyrights. They are delightful persons and are creating a new variety show.

    3:41 pm. I took a nap in Sam's office and feel much better – silent snores snap slow synapses.

Chapter Thirty-Seven
May 4, 2006

2:07 a.m. I rode my bike home last night and left my Parkinson's drugs at the office. I have tried to make Dragon Speak work but the program keeps crashing so I am slowly tapping out these words on my wireless keyboard held in my lap as I sit in the blue office chair at the foot of my bed. I cannot sell this loft; I need to figure out a way to keep it whether it is as rehearsal space or office space for the theater or otherwise. That may be the solution.

Forty-Five minute ago I spoke to Mara. It was the best conversation we have had in awhile but still ended up with her needing me to give her something; there was no I want to repay you for all the times I got money and said I would pay you back. She wants to have dinner tomorrow night and I am to bring the title to my Jeep Cherokee which looks great now that the body shop has fixed all the dents and dings and touched up the paint. Mara put in the sound system that I bought for at Best Buy with the last few hundred dollars of credit on my MBNA card. Mara said she needs to have title to the truck so she doesn't get in trouble with the law. I joked, "So are you going to dump now that you got everything you wanted?" She defended herself despite my comment that I was just joking. "I am not a gold digger," she said. "I just want to get everything in order. And I need to be able to say what I am thinking to you just like you do to me." I suspect she was thinking, "I need stability in knowing I have a vehicle and that you are not going to do what you did at Racine's and take the truck back by having Rachel steal it." I knew that was on her mind because of her text message to me when I encountered the barricaded door. Oddly it was the last text message she has sent me. It said, "Lemme kno when you wanna take my truck back lmao…Your confused."

We had a conversation earlier this evening while she was at Home Depot getting chain for the erotic swing that she had me buy at the Crypt, when she asked if I had the loft on the market yet and when I said no and that I was thinking of using it as rehearsal space as the theater she said, "I hate it when we talk about doing something and then I just hear that something else is happening."

Oh and the other thing she wants me to bring to the dinner is the print out of Fifty and Change – this writing. So like all books disclosed too soon there becomes the real possibility that review of others affects the writing –sort of like re-looping sound. But I shall focus on the events and try to describe them accurately, no matter what the consequence. I am sure all who read these words critically whether it is my Mistress or my editor or my readers will have their points of contention. Hopefully the re-looping does not create destructive reverberations. Perhaps I need to inquire of our rocket scientist client.

A new case for a scared woman and I suddenly see that practicing law has endless possibilities which is the same thing that the engineer Frank said to me yesterday. He said every job seems the same until he starts the project. We meet Friday and I sign off on a contract. Hopefully, I have the lease signed by then.

Tomorrow I meet with a ballet group about using the new theater. I told Mara that and told her I took ballet in college with my college girlfriend. I don't think we were hooked up at the time I took the class though later we were.

I definitely was naïve in college. Perhaps I still am.

I need more blueberry juice. I think Trevor's remedy is helping the Parkinson's effects because I am typing, albeit slowly.

Looking back at a journal again I see evidence of Parkinson's and evidence of my desire to write about what I see on a day-to-basis.

An entry from November 29, 2000, six months before I was diagnosed with Parkinson's. I was traveling on a case. The handwriting was very small.

Wed. 11/29/00

Headed for Cincinnati. When I carry heavy bags it is hard to scribble afterwards.

Now I'm on the plane in flight. It's dark outside and the engines hum and vibrate my seat. (I almost copied "seat" as "soul" I guess I have become more poetic these days.) Far below I see lights of a small town.

I had a black cab driver who took me from the hotel to the airport. He told me stories of his being a psychiatrist and comforter to a girl whose boyfriend liked cocks rather than her (he said she was so beautiful it would make your cock hard). She had been crying when she got in the car.

The cab driver told me he wasn't going to work hard anymore; he usually makes $300 a night. He said he just got his license back and gave me a precise date—September 23. He started driving then. He said cab driving was great; drug dealers would give him $20 for a $4 dollar ride—he said he got free drugs—cocaine and weed and sex from them too. He told me, as we pulled up to the airport about how a girl had blown him all the way and he kept making right turns one block from their destination till he came.

The writing went on and contrasted two persons. I am not sure if it was the same day or the next morning.

Morning Pages. Yesterday, on the flight from Cincinnati to Harrisburg, I sat next to an older lady with perfectly coiffed silver hair and glasses who was returning from Florida. She had visited a friend who had just turned 100. She was from Hershey, Pennsylvania and worked for Hershey Chocolate—I didn't know that's where the name had come from. She has a cat and agreed it is easier to leave a cat than a dog.

The cab driver told me his girlfriend does not like to give head and likes it when he goes down on her and then he fucks the hell out of her.

The cab driver was stocky but not tall and had a black stubble that darkened his already dark face.

The woman from Hershey sat next to me in the back of the plane and pointed out Three Mile Island Nuclear plant. She said, "Remember when we didn't know if it would blow up or not." In that comment and in her fascination with seeing the facility from the air I realized that she had suffered the stress of not knowing what would happen many years ago.

Now I have to get some more sleep because it is 3:45 a.m. and I have a huge day ahead of me. I am giving away my truck tomorrow, meeting with a Ballet company, finishing the theater lease and trying to perform magic for a new friend in need. I close with a quote from Tennessee Williams' forward to "A Streetcar Named Desire" that has driven me for years:

What is good? The obsessive interest in human affairs, plus a certain amount of compassion and moral conviction, that first made the experience of living something that must be translated into pigment or music or bodily movement or poetry or prose or anything that's dynamic and expressive—that's what's good for you if you're at all serious in your aims. William Saroyan wrote a great play on this theme, that purity of heart is the one success worth having. "In the time of your life—live!" That time is short and it doesn't return again. It is slipping away while I write this and while you read it, and the monosyllable of the clock is Loss, Loss, Loss, unless you devote your heart to its opposition.

Chapter Thirty-Eight
May 5, 2006

3:00 a.m. Last night I left the office around 6:45 p.m. drove south on I-25 to I-225 to the Iliff exit where I met Mara for dinner. She picked the place, Texas Steakhouse, one of the restaurants she later referred to as her "suburban ghetto" restaurants. She was ready on time, arriving a few minutes after I did. She was dressed in a short denim skirt and a low cut sleeveless black blouse with a purple and gray Playboy jacket and heels so high that she stood taller than me. She was gorgeous and I told her so several times. I had printed out Fifty and Change through yesterday's entry and I gave her a copy with the title to the Jeep Cherokee signed over to her. At the end of dinner, over my ineffectual protests, we went to American Furniture Warehouse and ordered 2,100 dollars worth of furniture payable in six months. What won me over was the fact that we ordered for us a table for the house so we can have romantic dinners. We also ordered a dresser which has a marble top and was on sale for $798 reduced from $1941 dollars. She has to put it in the living room because her huge bed and armoire fills her bedroom.

Back to dinner. I can see almost every moment from sitting down with her and drinking iceless "frozen" strawberry daiquiris to getting a to-go box for most of her dinner.

I executed the formalities of giving her the script and title quickly while we waited for the table. I warned her she might not like the story but that it was the truth. Later in the night, after we had dinner I told her that I wanted to use her photographs in the book.

However, dinner was not a "blonde-bombshell" discussion. Mara told me about her anger with her mother telling others that she had abandoned her family when in fact her mother had manipulated the system by manipulating her thirteen year old daughter. Mara told how the police were ready to arrest her mom for child abuse and then her mom figured out with her friends that if she said Mara had run away she would not be prosecuted.

Mara contrasted what happened to Alice's mother who had Alice at age 13 to what has happened to Mara. Alice's mother evidently is a drug addict and prostitute and failed to make the transition. Mara sees her life now as wonderful with endless possibilities. May I say with hope, she sees our lives as wonderful with endless possibilities. Mara has steel in her make-up that allows her not only be a dominatrix, but to be quietly sure of herself and her identity.

Mara told me that one of the things she is thankful for is that her heart is still open that she can still trust people. Or I suppose as Trevor would say she still believes in the Yellow Brick Road and that if you click your heels you still can go back to Kansas. As I write this I am crying. Last night when she told me about her heart I read her my quote from Tennessee Williams *"purity of heart is the one success worth having. "In the time of your life—live!"* and tears came to my eyes.

I never have felt more certain of our relationship than last night. As she drove me to American Furniture Warehouse in "her" truck she turned up the new stereo that has been installed. She laughed as I had to put my hands over my ears. The bass thump is amazing—a girl who knows stereos. I love her. I believe her when she tells me she loves me. I am happy walking around a furniture store with her.

One of the questions in my life may have been answered with my dinner with Mara. We talked about setting the wedding date this fall.

It is 4:30 a.m. and I am going running. Every day from now on I must focus on 175, thirty miles a week and published. It used to be that the first two goals and third hard, but somehow things have reversed. The first two are as essential as the third and much harder to attain right now.

Mara has some amazing fashion show ideas for the Blues House Theater. Will the theater be created? Can I get the lease signed today or Monday? Can I get enough money to pull off this feat or not because as Mara says once the theater is up and running we can make money.

Chapter Thirty-Nine
May 6, 2006

I thought about writing the word "disappointments" at the start of this Chapter and then write about all the disappointments I felt yesterday, but thankfully I did not. Rather I write about the amazingly good things that happened yesterday, including seeing an actor, the former theater company leader who moved to L.A. to make it as an actor and getting a email joke from a dead pan real estate broker. And writing poetry at the Mercury Café while I waited to read. I didn't get to the Mercury until 10:45 p.m. and almost had a horrendous car accident that would have been my fault and a direct result of talking on the cell to Mara while driving. Thank the heavens for allowing me to hit the breaks in time. It would be ironic to give away the Cherokee to Mara only to have my Wrangler destroyed and perhaps me with it.

So I wrote three poems while sitting next to a poet friend and read them at 12:30 a.m. at the Mercury with only a few persons still sitting there. They were well-applauded and audience members thanked me. I was thrilled at continuing my string of writing poems on the nights I signed up to read.

As I was writing the above paragraph, at 4:15 a. m. Mara called because she had seen that I had called. She said she had fallen asleep earlier and I know she was suffering from menstrual cramps and had been in pain and grumpy. Her voice was clear now as she told me that she loved me. I love her and any money issues I had earlier were washed away with the sweetness of her voice.

Before she went back to bed I read her the poems I wrote and read at the Mercury Café a few hours ago.

Shadowed chains restrain
The music of the cellos,
Purple words invoking clouds
Of pain,
Faces upturned into acid rain,
Tears falling forever,
To the sea,
Till green merges to red,
Red to blue,
Blue to Black,
And silence comes.

The second poem was also untitled:

Flowered petal pink
Never seems to sink,
In the washing, weeping waves
Bobbing in the ray
Of cloud focused sun
Till wooden dories draws near
And naïve young hand harvests
The soft pink rose
Riding the waves.

The third poem had a title:

Night Poet

Angles, Curves, Words,
Climbing, Sliding, Listening,
Legs, Asses, mouths,
Lego toys built of word dreams,
Rhymes, Times and verse,
Drink the flavored water daily,
Then say your prayers gently,
Till the poetry combines
The Curves and Rhymes, Angles and dreams,
Asses and times, Toys and words,
Thus relations unknown,
Each night are discovered,
 alone.

7:02 a.m. I just wrote a poem for a new post on my blog.

Once again I dabble as I am able
With blank page flat on the table,
Words affixed like gobs of paint.
Today, will me smear words with the taint
Of oily grifters not saints?
Or rather, shall I brush chalk
Of different colors for each who talks?
Watery images make mountains sag
When their outlines I clean

with my multicolored rag.
Yes, today I play with words,
And paint in black and white,
Made colorful by my readers imagination,
Not sight.

Chapter Forty
Sunday May 7, 2006

9:11 AM. I slept poorly night; I ate too much yesterday and did not work out. No work done and Mara called to see me at Target where she spent $560 in groceries and asundries. I use my credit card which has little left on it to buy groceries. And then I give Mara $300 cash. Strange how sometimes I feel used and other times in love. I guess I woke up unsettled. I have to stop by Nora house, Greg's friend, for breakfast; she wanted to cook for us. She wants to direct plays and be involved in the theater. As Mara said, "Why isn't anyone putting up any money but you?" Used! Go run and come back and see how you feel.

I can't even find my watch so I think I won't go anywhere. That is angry. I have to meet the needs of others that I cannot even anticipate. This anger will pass, but I hate it when it comes, the rage from lack of sleep and obligations I struggle to meet.

Today I feel the heavy clatter

Of obligations shoveled on my head,

Like clods of barely moist soil

Tumbling six feet to the dead,

Piling unorganized on the door

From which you exit no more.

Except the never heard dirt

Merely blankets your sleep

And today I'm awake

And my headache extends to my feet.

2:00 PM. I just got back to the office from over to Nora Woodard's house, a teacher at ooooooooooooooooooooooooooooooooooooooooooooooooooooooooooooooo]]a local college. She is a good friend of gregss Damn Parkinson's. I ate breakfast with Greg and sssssssssssssssssssssssssssssssssssssssssssssssssssssssssssssssssssssssssssssssssssssssssssssssssssssssssssssssssssssssssssssssssssssssssssssssssssssssssssss]]iiiiiiiiiiiiiiiiiiiiiiiiiiiiiiiiiiiiiiiiiiiiiiiiiiiiiiiiiiiiiiiiiiiiiiiiiiiiiiiiiiiiiiiiiiiiiiiiiiiiiiiiiiiiiiiiiiiiiiiiiiiiiiiiiiiiiiiiiiiiiiiiiiiiiiiiiiiiiiiiiiiooooooooooooo. I am exhausted, I took a copy of the script of aaaaaaaaaaaaaaaaaaaaaaaaaaaaaaaaaaaaaaaaaaaaaaaaaaaal[[[[[[[[[[[[[[[[[[[[[[[[[[[ss. I have to take a nap because I cannot work on the Complaint in this condition. My mind keeps shutting off and the fingers lock on the keyboard keys and the result is the long string of sssss's or aaaa's.

2:52PM. At the office. Now that I took a nap in the plush chair in Sam's office I am starting for real. I went to Nora's house andsssddddddddddddddddddddddddddddddddddddddddddddddddddddddddddddddddddddddddddddddddddddddddddddddddddddddddddddddddddddddddddddddd. Shit. Even with the nap I am having hard time writing. My mind keeps turning off and the keys are held down until the mind turns back on again. I have to work on the Complaint for the new case.

I have reached the end of Fifty and Change. On a strange impulse I printed and took this script with me to brunch and when Nora asked if I had anything to read I said I did but that it might shock them incredibly. She asked about what types of plays I wrote and I said, "This is really not a play." Greg asked, "Should we hear the writing first or eat first." I said, "Eat first." To myself I said, "And then we will see if I can read." For I was not certain that I could bring myself to read Fifty and Change to Greg and Nora. In fact it seemed unlikely to me that I would read anything but some poems.

We raucously discussed the merits of the production of Death of a Salesman that Greg and I had attended on Friday night. We agreed that Arthur Miller's writing was amazing and that the casting and direction was not. Greg and I both wanted to leave at intermission but we stayed to see our partner Jack scene whose role was all in the second act. After breakfast of delicious quiche and bagels and fruit, Nora ushered us out into the back yard. The sun was bright and she had a little platform with chairs and table set up by a head high wooden fence. Since she is a director and actor, I am sure many readings have occurred there.

When we sat down my heart was racing and my right hand trembling. I turned the script over when I had brought it in the house and I held it concealed as I took my seat in the back yard with Greg and Nora around the little low round table. I shuffled some pages from the back and was going to read the poems that I had written and read at the Mercury on Friday night after seeing "Death of a Salesman" with Greg. Then the moment came, the moment that has changed my life for all time. When the moment came I had no doubt. I put the pages back in order and began to read aloud Chapter One of Fifty and Change. When I looked up at the end of Chapter One and saw Greg and Nora both laughing and wiping away tears, I started to read Chapter Two.

www.ingramcontent.com/pod-product-compliance
Lightning Source LLC
Chambersburg PA
CBHW020911090426
42736CB00008B/578